Clinician's Guide to

Stages of Accomplishment Workbooks

For Sexually Abusive Youth in Treatment

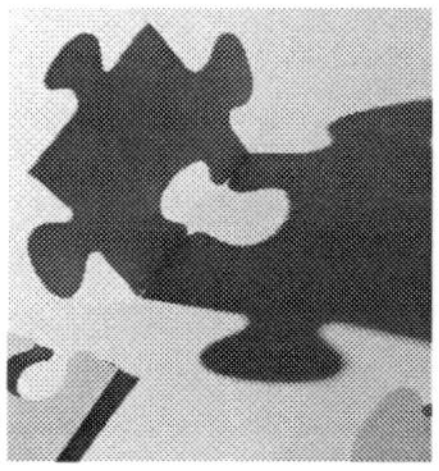
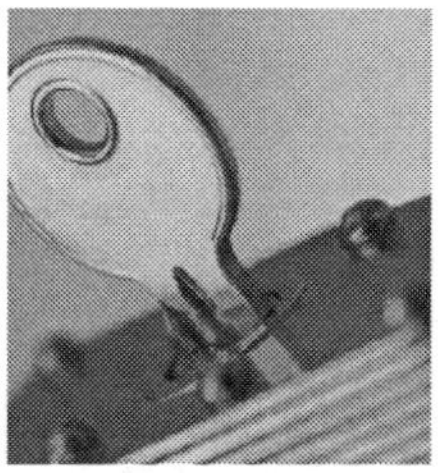
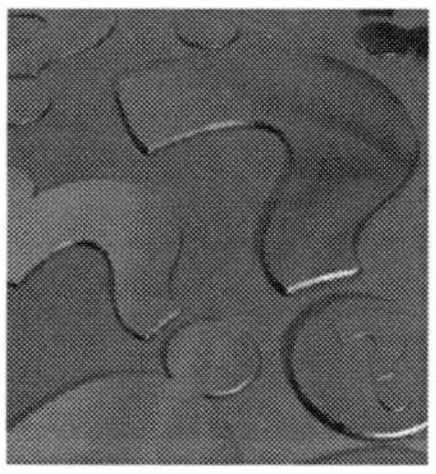
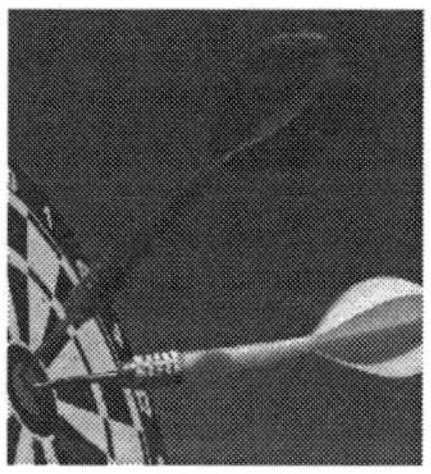

Phil Rich, Ed.D., MSW

Clinician's Guide to
Stages of Accomplishment Workbooks

Published by:
NEARI Press
70 North Summer Street
Holyoke, MA 01040
413.540.0712

Distributed by:
NEARI Distribution
10 Water Street
P.O. Box 1220
Lebanon, NH 02766
888.632.7412
ISBN# 978-1-929657-41-4

The Author

Phil Rich is the Clinical Director of Stetson School. He has worked with children, adolescents, and families for more than thirty years, and sees sexually troubled youth in just the same way as all of the other children and adolescents with whom he has worked – as valuable, important, and capable young people on a path than can lead to success and satisfaction, even though there are pitfalls along the way. It is the support, encouragement, guidance, and belief in their capacities, and in them, that often makes the difference. Phil presents and trains nationally and internationally, and is the author of several books that address the assessment and treatment of sexually abusive youth.

Contents

The Development of the *Stages of Accomplishment Workbooks*

The Stages of Accomplishment workbooks were developed for adolescents in treatment at Stetson School, a residential treatment program in Massachusetts that specializes in the treatment of sexually abusive and sexually inappropriate behavior in children and adolescent boys. Many pre-adolescent and adolescent boys have passed through Stetson School and have done remarkably well in our program and in every aspect of their post-residency lives. They came to realize that they are capable of a great deal of success, and the same is true for many, if not most, children and adolescents with sexual behavior problems. We know – and our treatment is based on that knowledge – that the youths with whom we work are far, far more than simply their sexually abusive or sexually inappropriate behavior.

Developed for and in use at Stetson School, these workbooks are used with other materials, including other workbooks, and are built into a treatment program that recognizes young people as "whole" people, and in which the ***relationship*** between youths and the staff who work with them is the central and perhaps most important feature of treatment. Workbooks are important, as are the ideas they teach and the self-discovery and change they promote; however, it is the relationships that are essential.

Although designed and developed at Stetson School, the ideas and materials are well-informed and developed in concert with the thinking in our field. Any workbook, including the four in this series, represents simply one element of treatment, as described in this *Clinician's Guide*. The ideas are far-ranging and may be used in any treatment program; they do not reflect methods, approaches, and/or philosophies unique to any single program or orientation to treatment.

Section I: Introduction

Introduction to the Clinician's Guide

This *Clinician's Guide* will help clinicians to use the *Stages of Accomplishment Workbooks* most effectively in their practice with individual clients and/or as a part of a larger treatment program. The *Guide* describes the ideas, practices, and models that underlie the workbooks. Through reading this *Guide,* clinicians will quickly become familiar with the workbooks as a whole as well as the structure and content of individual chapters.

Once familiar with the *Stages* workbooks, you will need little guidance in its use and will be able to adapt it to fit your own approach to the treatment of sexually abusive youth, or youths who engage in sexually troubled behavior. The *Clinician's Guide* will not only acquaint you with the workbooks as a whole, but also with the use of workbooks in general, and how to best use the workbooks as part of a larger program of and approach to treatment. It will also assist you in understanding how to select, assign, and use the written exercises and how to best use the Thinking Points, Key Concepts, and the general text, as well as understanding and facilitating each youth's general use of and experience with the workbooks.

Written to provide a strong resource, *The Clinician's Guide* is also designed to be accessible and simple to use. For this reason, the guide is divided into several sections for easy reference. Clinicians may choose to read the entire *Clinician's Guide*, or more simply review Section V of the Guide, which provides a detailed overview of the each of the Stages workbooks and their contents on a chapter-by-chapter basis.

The *Stages of Accomplishment Workbooks*

The four inter-related *Stages of Accomplishment Workbooks* are written for adolescent boys of low-average and above intelligence, whose primary language is English, and who have engaged in sexually abusive behavior, as well as sexually troubled and sexually inappropriate behavior even if not reaching a level of sexual abuse. These youths will be in residential care or in community treatment, although the most comprehensive use and utility of the workbooks is in conjunction with residential treatment or group care where treatment is usually more comprehensive and wrapped around almost all aspects of client lives during the course of such treatment.

Although designed for adolescent boys of average intelligence, the workbooks can be used with or adapted for different populations, including younger children, cognitively lower functioning individuals, and girls. These treatment populations represent a different "audience" for whom, in some cases, workbook content, required reading and comprehension level, and treatment concepts may be too complex, do not apply, or are clearly aimed at a different target population. Adaptations and alternative materials for different populations are discussed and described below, with some considerations for such use.

Why "Stages of Accomplishment"?

The "Stages of Accomplishment" model was developed as a means both to teach the treatment concepts and engagement we wanted to foster in our clients and to provide a means of recognition when our clients showed acquisition, retention, and application of those concepts.

The model was designed as a means for youths to demonstrate and be recognized for their accomplishments in learning, not as a measure of treatment "success" or treatment "progress," or as a "level-and-privilege" system. With the accomplishment of each stage, the youths with whom we work are thus able to show themselves, their families, and others that they are learning important ideas about treatment, and are able to use these ideas in their everyday life.

Incorporating Workbooks as One Element of Treatment

As described in Section III of this *Guide* under "Workbook Completion Time," "workbook completion" does not equal "treatment completion," whether the workbooks are used as adjuncts to treatment or as the basis for a structured and sequenced program of treatment."

It is particularly important that workbook use, assignment, and completion be treated as one element among others that contribute to reflect participation and growth when used within a larger treatment program. In such a model, it is ***more*** important to have consistent improvements in behaviors, social interactions, and psychosocial functioning provide evidence of treatment participation, the internalization of treatment ideas, and personal growth rather than just the completion of workbooks. Workbook use should not be rushed; but regardless of how quickly or slowly they are completed, alone they do not provide evidence of real change.

Brief Outline of the *Stages of Accomplishment Workbooks* and Chapters

Each of the four workbooks in the Stages of Accomplishment series is built in an inter-related sequence. Moving from more basic and less intensive material to more complex and detailed material and work, each workbook builds the foundation for the following workbook or builds upon the foundation set by the prior workbook. Although each workbook can be used as a "stand alone" element of treatment, the series was designed to be used together and in sequence.

A brief description of each workbook, by title and chapter, is provided below. A more detailed description can be found in Section V of this *Guide*, more specifically familiarizing clinicians with the content and use of the workbooks on a chapter-by-chapter basis.

Workbook 1. *An Introduction to Treatment*

Youths learn about treatment, and about themselves and why they are're in treatment. The workbook covers ideas and information about sexually abusive and sexually inappropriate behavior.

Chapter 1. Introduction to Treatment
Chapter 2. Participating in Your Treatment
Chapter 3. Understanding Sexually Abusive Behavior

Workbook 2. *Understanding Yourself*

Youths learn more about themselves, including their feelings, attitudes, and ideas, and how these responses can come together to contribute to sexually abusive or sexually inappropriate behavior.

Chapter 1. Learning About Yourself
Chapter 2. Feelings, Thoughts, and Behaviors
Chapter 3. Understanding and Managing Feelings
Chapter 4. Attitudes, Beliefs, and Values
Chapter 5. Thinking Errors

Workbook 3. *Understanding Dysfunctional Behavior*

The *Stage 3 Workbook* helps youths to understand their problematic behaviors, and the impact of their behavior on others.

Chapter 1. Dysfunctional Behavioral Cycles
Chapter 2. Phases of the Dysfunctional Behavioral Cycle
Chapter 3. High-Risk Situations and Behaviors
Chapter 4. Behavior Management, Staying Safe, and Preventing Relapse

Workbook 4. *Hitting the Target: Making Permanent Change*

The final workbook in the series helps youths learn how to better understand and connect with others and their community, make amends for their sexually abusive or inappropriate behavior, relate and give back to their community, and build stronger relationships with others.

Chapter 1. Thinking About Others: Empathy and Caring
Chapter 2. Victim Awareness and Clarification
Chapter 3. Community Service
Chapter 4. Learning to Communicate
Chapter 5. Healthy Relationships
Chapter 6. Epilogue: Your Final Words

Sexual Offender-Specific Treatment/Sexually Troubled Behavior

We've already referred to sexually inappropriate and sexually troubled behavior, in addition to sexually abusive behavior. However, it's clear from the titles of the workbooks that their primary target is youth with sexually abusive behaviors, rather than a more general group of youths who demonstrate sexually troubled behavior.

Nevertheless, we recognize that adolescents whose sexual behaviors are of concern, but who have not reached a level where they have become (or are not known to have become) sexually abusive also enter treatment, sometimes in the same treatment programs that treat sexually abusive behavior. Therefore, the workbooks are designed to also help in providing treatment for this sub-morbid, or "sub-legal-threshhold," population of sexually *troubled*, but not sexually *abusive*, adolescents.

Language and Labeling

We have addressed ideas and concerns about labeling children and adolescents in the Stages of Accomplishment workbooks directly. We hope that we have done so with sensitivity and objectivity, with the goal of helping youths in treatment to both understand the labels that are applied to their behaviors and to them, and to allow youths to move beyond such labels, no matter what form they may take. We wish to help these youths recognize and work through their problematic behaviors but also experience and understand themselves as whole people with a range of strengths and skills, and not simply as sexually abusive adolescents.

You, as the clinician, must decide for yourself ***your*** choice of language, from "juvenile sexual offender" to "sexually abusive youth" to "adolescents with sexual behavior problems," and more. We recommend that you discuss these labels and terms with your clients, thus helping them recognize and deal with the range of labels, no matter what they may be, that are attached to them as a result of their behavior.

Our Clients Are Whole People

Beyond labels, and far beyond the subject of sexually abusive behavior addressed in these workbooks, we recognize and respond to the children, adolescents, and young people with whom we work as whole people, in which sexually abusive behavior or other forms of sexually troubled behavior represent simply one element of their makeup and experience.

The *Stages* workbooks deal with many issues faced and experienced by youths who engage in sexually abusive behavior. It is a central tenet of the Stages of Accomplishment model that our clients are whole people, that sexually abusive and sexually inappropriate behavior must and can only be understood and treated in this context, and that this idea must be imparted to the youths with whom we work, their families, other providers who provide treatment and care, and the community at large.

A Note on Pronouns

As noted, the *Stages of Accomplishment* workbooks are designed and intended for use with adolescent boys. Accordingly, male pronouns, such as "he" or "his," are typically used when a gender-specific reference is made. However, because the workbooks can, with caution and sensitivity, be used and adapted for use with girls, a "she" or "her" is occasionally dropped into the text, reminding the clinician of the possibility that the workbooks may be used with both males and females. The periodic use of female pronouns also serves to remind clinicians that, although a predominately male crime, sexually abusive behavior is not necessarily limited to males.

Section II: The Application and Approach of the Workbooks

Applying the Stages Workbooks in the Larger Treatment Environment

The *Stages* workbooks were designed to help youths both learn new information and use the workbooks as a therapeutic tool intended to help them think about, work through, and address important elements in their treatment and in their lives, including as a means for self-reflection. Through the written exercises and Thinking Points, the workbooks provide a means for self-discovery and the learning and practicing of new skills in self-awareness. These exercises and Thinking Points vary in content and approach, and different exercises are intended for different purposes in the therapeutic process.

Part of the art and skill of therapy lies in knowing when and how to help clients tackle the issues they are facing. Accordingly, clinicians using the *Stages* workbooks must be familiar enough with the outline of the workbooks, their approach, the information contained within each workbook, and the written exercises and Thinking Points in sufficient detail to know when they're likely to be useful, when the client is ready to meaningfully tackle the work, when to repeat an exercise or assignment, and even when the completion of certain material is not likely to be productive at that point in treatment or may even be counter-productive. Once you are familiar with the *Stages* workbooks, you'll adapt them to your own theoretical approach and style.

Your use of the *Stages* workbooks will be influenced by many factors: the treatment location (outpatient, residential care, inpatient, intensive outpatient treatment, etc.), the ability of each youth to work on specific and often increasingly difficult material, the client's progress and participation in therapy, and the stage in therapy, to name but a few variables. Under any treatment condition, however, workbooks serve as a valuable adjunct. The need to extend treatment outside of the boundaries of the therapist's office or the treatment program makes the use of the workbook still more important.

If the ultimate goal of all therapy is to help clients learn to do without the therapist, then your use of the Stages workbooks has still more value, as it makes it clear in your work with your clients that the journey is *theirs*. By making this case clear to clients from the outset, you increase the chances that your clients will eventually be able to continue on their journey under their own direction.

The Approach of the Workbooks

As is true for many workbooks, the *Stages of Accomplishment Workbooks* provide a primarily psychoeducational approach to treatment. In treatment, psychoeducation involves an instructional approach to teaching clients concepts, tools, methods, and/or skills considered important to their treatment and rehabilitation.

However, the workbooks also provide a means for both self-guided learning and self-discovery, and the integration of ideas and experience. As an adjunct to treatment, the workbooks also serve as a foundation for and extension of interactive, face-to-face counseling or psychotherapy through which their ideas can be brought to life and explored and developed in a manner that psychoeducation alone can never hope to accomplish.

Using the Stages Workbooks: Standardized and Individualized Treatment

The principle upon which these workbooks is built is that they add to a model of treatment that is far greater than the material in the workbooks itself, and that treatment should and must be individualized to each client.

Because sexual offender-specific treatment is substantially different from other forms of treatment, aimed at substantially different treatment targets, it is reasonable to consider it essential to have a set of standardized ideas and tools that represent its core elements. The *Stages* workbooks help to fill that need, and can be used as the basis for a structured model of treatment that includes standardized elements, follows a standardized sequence, and provides a standardized core for a program of treatment, while helping to ensure that treatment is delivered in an individualized manner and is customized for each individual client.

The *Stages* workbooks can help ensure that clinicians, while individualizing treatment, are also tightly focused on the sexually abusive and sexually troubled aspects of client behavior. That is, they are teaching and discussing with their clients common ideas and tools that are specific to such behavior, and teaching a common language to clients, and furthermore to the ***families*** of clients if they are included in treatment (which we strongly encourage and, frankly, would expect in a well-developed and comprehensive program of treatment).

Although standardized in content and design, the workbooks can be adapted in many ways to meet the needs and goals of individualized treatment, including the needs of different youths at particular points in their treatment. This customization largely involves how they are actually used by different clinicians, in the choice of reading and workbook exercises that clinicians assign to individual clients, in the sequencing of workbook use, and in adding to and going beyond the material in the workbooks.

It is not a difficult task to have a standardized treatment model serve as the basis for a treatment program that is also individualized. A standard model builds upon a "core" program through which all clients pass, teaching general ideas about sexually abusive and sexually troubled behavior to all clients, and will perhaps assess treatment progress on the basis of standardized expectations. On the other hand, an individualized model of treatment is geared to the needs of individual clients and individual circumstances, addressing and treating not only matters related to sexually problematic behavior but also treatment needs that go far beyond the sexually abusive or troubled behavior itself and are idiosyncratic to each individual client.

"Manualization" and Workbooks

The four workbooks, as an integrated whole, do not add up to a treatment "manual" and should not be considered or used as such. A treatment manual typically not only describes elements and steps of treatment, but prescribes treatment and usually requires that the clinician follow the steps and ideas of the manual, and what is often the single theoretical approach endorsed by the manual. Treatment manuals can be rigid, and often, even if not always, add up to a "one-size-fits-all" or "recipe" approach to the treatment of all clients. Manuals also often eliminate, or seriously dampen, clinical flexibility and certainly the ability to individualize not just treatment itself, but the clinician's *approach* to treatment. A manualized approach to treatment implies, and usually requires, a single approach, a prescribed sequence, and a regimented application to treatment and defines the elements that comprise treatment. The *Stages* workbooks are not manuals. They are, instead, "workbooks," designed to assist and add to treatment rather than define, drive, or "methodologize" treatment and the treatment process.

The Benefits of Workbooks

Workbooks can and, if used well, ***will*** extend treatment beyond the confines of a clinician's office, beyond group treatment, and beyond time-bound elements of treatment such as the therapy session or a time- and frequency-limited set of therapy sessions. Workbooks can be used to extend the ideas discussed and taught in individual, group, and family therapy sessions, and can be used to prepare clients for planned sessions that are yet to happen. They can be used to discuss ideas, provide information, explore situations, and teach skills, and can do so in ways that are frankly not otherwise possible, often due to time restraints, but for other reasons as well.

To this degree, workbooks are akin to academic homework, although they need not necessarily be assigned this way, in that they extend teaching (the teacher's task) and learning (the student's task) outside of the classroom. Workbooks provide an alternate means for students to acquire and retain information, augment classroom education and provide more time for learning, and additionally place a level of responsibility on the student for engagement in the learning process. Homework also allows, to some degree, self-paced learning, questions-and-answers that cannot be addressed (or even necessarily thought of) in the classroom, and an objective means for recognizing not simply the comprehension and acquisition of information but also the student's level of motivation and engagement in the learning process.

However, nobody would seriously consider replacing classroom and individualized teaching with homework. In fact, it is clear that homework extends and is based upon classroom instruction, and does not represent "stand alone" or "replacement" education. Even if people can learn from homework and independent study (which they clearly can), in this context homework extends, but does not replace, face-to-face education.

So it is with the *Stages* workbooks. They extend teaching and learning, exploration, experimentation, self-discovery, and the development of insight and awareness far beyond the therapist's office. They allow ideas that have been discussed and tools that have been taught to be further explored and developed after and between sessions, and they allow clients to explore and be prepared to discuss ideas and tools ahead of sessions planned to cover such material. In some cases, workbooks may cover material that will not be covered in individual sessions at all, other than through a brief review of the material and how well the client has completed workbook assignments. Workbooks can not only *extend* therapy beyond and between sessions, they can also be used to prepare clients *for* therapy, explaining the therapeutic process and how best to engage in and use the process.

Workbooks can be used to teach information and ideas, engage clients in self-discovery, prepare clients for further discussion, and develop a knowledge and skill base in clients. Workbooks can be used to test for comprehension and for the depth of comprehension and acquisition. In addition, the use (and completion) of workbooks holds clients responsible, at least in part, for their participation in treatment, and allows clinicians to assess the motivation of clients to engage in treatment, and how far such motivation goes.

Workbooks also maintain a permanent record of information taught, the acquisition of such information, and the depth of learning. They can be re--visited and serve to refresh memory over time, and workbooks tasks and exercises can be re--assigned as deemed necessary or relevant to any given situation or client. Workbooks also allow others who have legitimate access to treatment records and materials, who are not otherwise directly related to individual treatment, to gain insight into material taught, client exploration and comprehension, and client motivation and participation.

Workbook Limitations

There a number of potential limitations inherent to workbooks and their use.

Despite your best efforts, for instance, workbooks can homogenize and give treatment the appearance of being one-size-fits-all. Furthermore, many clients can "successfully" complete workbook materials without actually learning anything, or without incorporating any real change into their thinking or behavior. There is a risk, for instance, that rather than acquiring, understanding, and internalizing change, the completion of workbooks will actually help some clients to simply mimic true understanding, or "parrot" back information that makes it appear that they "get it," when in reality they don't get it at all. Additionally, workbooks can be completed casually and carelessly, and sometimes the "answer" to a particular question or exercise is obvious and can thus be completed easily without any real gain.

Furthermore, there is the risk, endemic to all workbooks, that clients don't complete the homework at all or hurry through assignments, completing them in the most minimal of ways, and in the process learn little if anything at all. In still other cases, workbook material may go right over the heads of some youths for any number of reasons, including developmental level, cognitive ability, learning style, language skill, and cultural background. Many youths, for example, may require a different or more carefully explained approach than can be managed by the workbook.

Related to these concerns, the best and most effective use of the *Stages* workbooks requires time for clinicians to review and understand their content before use. And as all teachers know, any assigned homework requires time – which in many programs may be in short supply – to review and evaluate the student's level of understanding. Without reviewing and re--visiting the material covered in workbooks and usually completed through homework assignments, workbook material may ***never*** be discussed during individual or group sessions or integrated into the larger treatment programs. Worse, there may be an unwarranted assumption that the material has been learned, retained and integrated when, in fact, it has not. This tendency is always a risk to be aware of and guard against in using workbooks.

Workbooks are also, of course, finite and limited in space. They always have a beginning and an end, and when they contain written exercises there is space to complete each exercise only once. This structure can create the illusion that once completed – that is, when all of the pages have been read and all of the exercises completed once – the work has been completed. This, however, is not true. The workbook is not ***the*** treatment, and the completion of the workbook neither represents the end of treatment nor the end of the utility of the workbook itself. Nevertheless, the physical limitations of workbooks represent an inherent problem that suggests that workbook completion somehow equals content mastery and perhaps even the completion of treatment, or at least that portion of the treatment.

Fitting the Workbook to the Treatment Program

One additional, and potentially significant, problem is that some workbook material may not fit with the ideas, or even the sensibilities, of different clinicians or different treatment programs, or diverges from the materials and ideas taught by clinicians and treatment programs.

The risks are that the workbooks will be used in a disjointed manner, that some workbook material may be completely eliminated, that treatment will get wrapped around the workbooks in a way that may not fit with the clinician or treatment program's model, or that workbook material and ideas presented in treatment simply don't fit together or are different. Accordingly, it is important to ensure an integrated fit between workbooks and the larger treatment model into which workbook use is embedded. It is particularly important that workbooks do not drive treatment, or become the "tail that wags the dog."

Accordingly, clinicians and treatment programs that use workbooks must figure out how to adapt their treatment models to fit the workbooks' approach and ideas or how to use workbooks so that they best fit the approach and ideas of the treatment program.

10 Pointers for Best Use

These 10 pointers, presented in alphabetical order, will both help overcome the limitations of workbooks and maximize their value.

Be selective and judicious. Don't feel compelled to use all of the material or ideas in the *Stages* workbooks if they do not fit with other materials or ideas you use. However, if material is by--passed or eliminated, take into consideration how or whether this will affect the completion of other workbook material.

Bring ideas and materials to life. Use discussion, explanation, illustration, reflection, and examples to bring the content of workbook assignments to life, helping to ensure not just clarification but relevance and depth of meaning.

Complete workbook assignments in therapy sessions. At times, complete workbook assignments with your client during therapy sessions. Working on assignments together, at least on occasion, can help bring material to life, help clients learn how to best use workbooks, work through difficult areas, and allow you to see the client's understanding and use of the workbooks in "action."

Customize treatment. Individualize your use of the workbooks so that it recognizes and meets the treatment needs of each client and the needs of treatment at any given point in time.

Expand upon the workbooks. Don't allow the fact the workbook is finite, with limited space and exercises that are provided only once, to limit your use of it. Workbook exercises, for instance, can be repeated, and reading material and content can be re--assigned as appropriate. Of equal value, clinicians can easily extend workbook exercises and content by creating and adding their own written exercises and additional material.

Go beyond the boundaries of the workbooks. Don't stop at the boundaries of the workbooks. Expand upon them, build upon their ideas, and develop new ideas and materials.

Integrate and blend material. Integrate the workbooks with your own ideas and approaches, and with other prepared materials thatn you may use in treatment.

Repeat and re–visit. Whenever necessary or it seems appropriate have clients go back to earlier workbook sections or material, either because they did not previously show a full understanding of or commitment to the ideas, or because those previous materials take on new meaning in your client's current point in treatment or under current circumstances in your client's life.

Review, discuss, and test for retention and comprehension. Review the manner in which youths use the workbooks and complete assignments, and discuss this with clients. Through review and discussion, ensure that clients complete exercises, retain knowledge, and demonstrate understanding of the material. Can clients, for instance, apply learned ideas to real life situations, interactions, and circumstances? (Brief tests for each workbook are provided in Appendix G.)

Show interest. Beyond reviewing and discussing the workbooks simply to ensure they are completed, show interest in the work your clients are completing, by reading their materials, listening to their ideas and their experiences with those ideas, asking additional questions, and answering any questions that your clients may have.

Working at the Client's Level

Because the workbooks are standardized, they are necessarily written for a projected "standard" youth – a male adolescent ranging between low-average to above-average intelligence, whose primary language is English. However, even within this range there is great variation, in age, cognitive development, intelligence, emotional maturity, language skills, social skill development, learning style, and sometimes in the client's primary language, as well as ethnic, cultural, and sub-cultural membership.

Accordingly, the clinician must recognize and take into account these many potential differences and ensure that the assignment and discussion of workbook material is aimed at the cognitive, developmental, skill, and psychological level of each individual client. This not only helps increase the chances that youths can and will understand and internalize the material and experience success, but is also a facet of individualizing treatment, and gearing treatment to the needs and capacities of each client.

Section III: Considerations in the Use of the *Stages of Accomplishment Workbooks*

Workbook Completion Time

We have stressed the relationship between the use and completion of workbooks and the larger treatment environment into which workbook use is incorporated, briefly discussed in Section I. From this perspective, it is unlikely that simply completing one or all of the workbooks will accomplish very much at all, other than perhaps the simple acquisition of information for some youths. And for some youths, that acquisition will soon fade into the background; even among those who retain the information, many will nevertheless not apply any of the information or incorporate it into their daily lives.

In fact, for youths who have a range of cognitive skills, and particularly those that relate to written material and instruction, these workbooks may be relatively easy to complete. For these youths, if they can sustain their attention, each workbook can be completed in a week or less. For other adolescents it may simply be impossible to finish the workbooks at all, due to attention difficulties, lack of comprehension, incapacity to sit still, limited cognitive skills, different learning styles or needs, or disinterest, lack of motivation, or plain boredom. The question, then, is not how long does it take to complete the workbooks, but how does the clinician use the workbooks in terms of assignments to ensure as best as possible that workbook material is not simply completed but actually learned, taken on-board, and applied?

In practice, treatment gains are judged by changes in behavior, self-regulation, social interactions, and improved psychosocial functioning, and not solely the completion of the workbooks. Recognizing, then, that workbooks can be completed quickly by some adolescents and very slowly by others, your use and assignment of workbooks should be guided by your goals in using workbooks; the skills, needs, and motivations, of your client; the venue and amount of time available for treatment; and the nature of available or relevant after-services in terms of post-discharge treatment follow up after you have discharged your client from treatment. It is entirely possible that your client will work on only one or two *Stages* workbooks while in treatment with you and may work on the remaining workbooks in treatment with his (or her) next provider if after-care treatment is provided.

Workbook completion is not to be rushed. Although a workbook ***can*** be completed in a few days, and certainly within a week, we suggest that at least two weeks be assigned for each workbook, with at least two weeks ***between*** workbooks, to be used for review, discussion, and re-visiting of workbook material and to assess any gains that seem to flow from workbook use. This represents a minimum of four weeks per workbook, including even the first and simplest and shortest workbook, for a total of 16 weeks for all four workbooks, or approximately four months.

However, it is more likely that these, and perhaps other workbooks as well, will be more effectively incorporated into treatment over a longer period of time, of perhaps at least six months duration. In fact, the more complex workbooks are likely to take three weeks to complete and perhaps more if, for instance, one chapter a week is assigned. Additionally, in a structured and longer-term treatment program in which there are often many treatment elements, such as those found in residential programs for example, it may be more useful to slow down the assignment of workbooks and spread out their use, along with other elements of treatment, over a longer period of time.

So, when all is said and done, workbook assignment and completion should range between a minimum of 4 months and, more productively and in a well-paced treatment environment, over a longer period of time, perhaps extending six to nine months into treatment.

Using the Stages Workbooks with Different Client Populations

The Stages workbooks are designed and intended for use with adolescent boys of average (or low-average) and higher intelligence, but may be adapted for use with different juvenile populations, such as children with sexual behavior problems, sexually abusive girls, and cognitively lower functioning juveniles. Just as each of these populations, as well as children and adolescents from different cultures and sub-cultures, differ from average intelligence adolescent boys, they are also quite different from one another.

Accordingly, if these workbooks are used with a population other than that for which they were designed, adjustments must be made to fit and adapt them for that ***particular*** population (teenage girls, for instance, versus pre-adolescent girls or cognitively impaired adolescents). The same is true to a great degree for youths whose primary language is not English, not simply because they may have difficulty with comprehension but because these youths may also have difficulty with concepts if they are culturally distinct from the English speaking adolescent boys who are the treatment target of these workbooks.

Many of the ideas and materials found in the *Stages of Accomplishment Workbooks* are appropriate and relevant to any teenager engaging in sexually abusive or troubled behavior, male or female, as well as many pre-adolescent children. The differences are most apparent in the manner in which the information and ideas are presented, the language and its level of complexity, and in some of the stories that illustrate ideas. Although workbook material may be adapted, the workbooks should be used with sensitivity with children and adolescents outside of the intended target population, and will need further customization.

With lower functioning adolescents, both language and concepts typically ***must*** be simplified. For pre-adolescent children, ideas must be simplified. The ideas and concepts about what drives sexualized behavior, and especially sexually abusive behavior, may not apply to the motivations and ideation of children. For pre-adolescent and adolescent girls and young women, different motivations and interests, as well as different social behaviors and social needs, apply rather than those described in the workbooks.

An Alternative to the Dysfunctional Behavioral Cycle

In working with lower cognitively functioning youths and pre-adolescents, and even with some average intelligence adolescents, it is possible to use a simpler model of the dysfunctional behavioral cycle, or a model that turns that "cycle" into something more linear and thus easier to follow for children and adolescents with less developed cognitive skills. The "One Safe Step at a Time" ("Safe Steps") model is shown in Appendix A, and Appendix B provides a simplified version of the dysfunctional behavioral cycle used in the Stages workbooks, designed in this case to be used with the Safe Steps model.

The simplified Safe Steps model illustrates one variation of the ideas and models used in the Stages workbooks. Although not used in either the workbooks or in this guide to the workbooks, it is also possible to simplify and create variants of the thinking errors and other tools and concepts described in the workbooks, designed specifically for developmentally less-sophisticated children and lower cognitively functioning adolescents.

On Behavioral Cycles and Relapse Prevention Plans

It is no surprise that behaviors are repetitive, including dysfunctional behaviors, as well as the thoughts and emotions that lie behind and drive behavior. Indeed, this is the basic premise of cognitive-behavioral therapies which aim to change behaviors and their emotional underpinnings by restructuring the ideation that influences, and sometimes drives, them both.

A behavioral cycle model is basic to any form of cognitive-behavioral therapy, even if referred to as something else. The basic A-B-C model of such therapy is a linear version of the behavioral cycle, and follows a simple pathway. Fundamental beliefs about self and others lead to automatic thoughts or cognitive responses, mediated by intermediate beliefs that involve attitudes and assumptions. Automatic thoughts, in turn, lead directly to emotional, physiological, and behavioral responses. That is, an **A**ctivating event leads to a rational or irrational **B**elief, that results in a **C**onsequence or behavioral outcome. In terms of the typical sex offender-specific version, the Activating event serves as the trigger to a Belief, or thinking error, which leads to a Consequence or outcome in the form of undesirable behavior, typically referred to as a relapse. The effects that follow the behavior serve as feedback of some kind, as shown simply in Figure 1, turning the linear model into a cyclical model that is often self-reinforcing, or in terms of behavioral therapy, builds a conditioned response that maintains a predictable and repetitive set of behaviors.

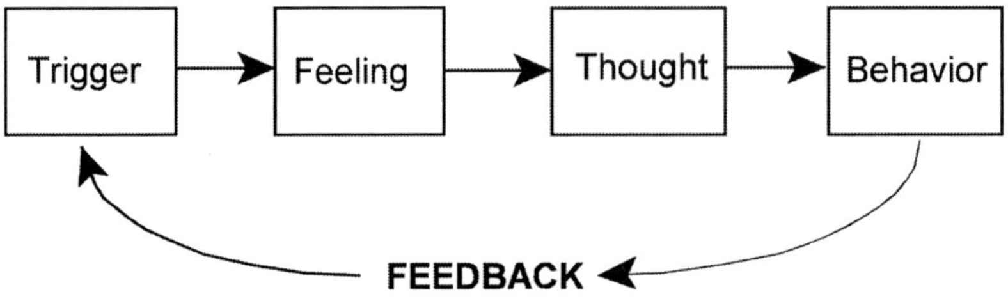

The behavioral cycle model has long been in use in the treatment of both adult and adolescent sexually abusive behavior, but has recently been examined with more care and more critically, as it should be (for example, see Letourneau & Borduin, 2008). Despite our more sophisticated and better informed apprehension of these models, they nevertheless continue to have great utility, and especially when used to depict and map out **any** form of repetitive dysfunctional behavior. In effect, cycles are predictions of trajectory – that is, the obvious path of a set of thoughts, feelings, and eventually behaviors if things continue as they always have. When it comes to negative and destructive behaviors, it is the job of treatment to intervene and change the direction and course of the typical trajectory.

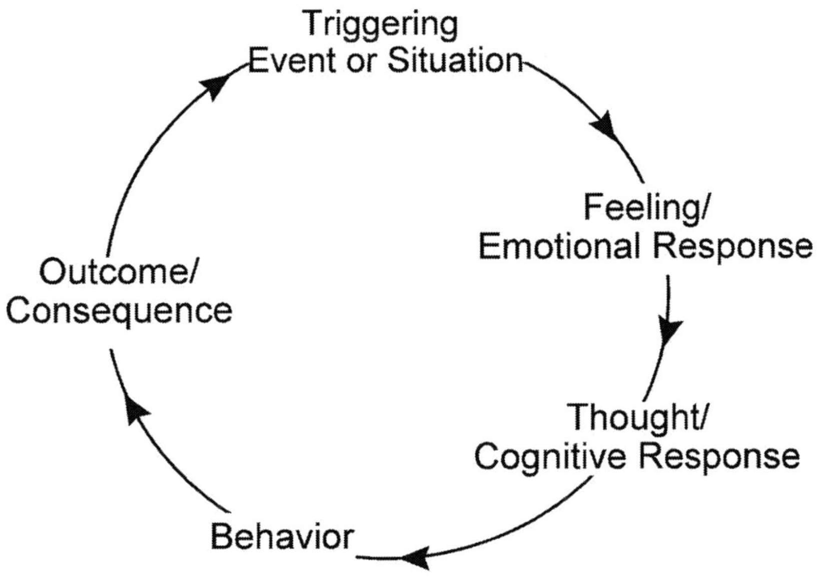

In the *Stages* workbooks, the cycle illustrated and taught is one of dysfunctional behaviors, shown in Figure 2. We do not use a model of the "sexual assault cycle," as it is sometimes called. The dysfunctional behavioral cycle may be used to describe and discuss repetitive sexually abusive behaviors or the possibility that sexually abusive behavior may recur, but this behavior is seen as one of many possible dysfunctional behaviors. A sexual assault cycle, on the other hand, assumes a more black-and-white model of behavior that is specific to sexually abusive behavior, and further that there has already been a *pattern* of such behavior (rather than simply one instance, for example).

A dysfunctional behavioral cycle is far broader and more generic and versatile with greater applicability. Further, the dysfunctional behavioral cycle model described in the *Stage* workbooks does not assume or assert that every individual who falls into dysfunctional behavior has the same experiences or experiences these behaviors in the same way. Instead, as described in the *Stage 3 Workbook*, and briefly in Section V of this *Clinician's Guide*, the cycle is visualized as occurring in sequential and predictable phases, as shown in Figure 3. Although individuals predictably pass through each phase en route to the next phase in the sequence, how long they remain in each phase and their experiences in each phase will vary widely based on the individual characteristics of different people and the circumstances in which the dysfunctional behavioral cycle develops and unfolds.

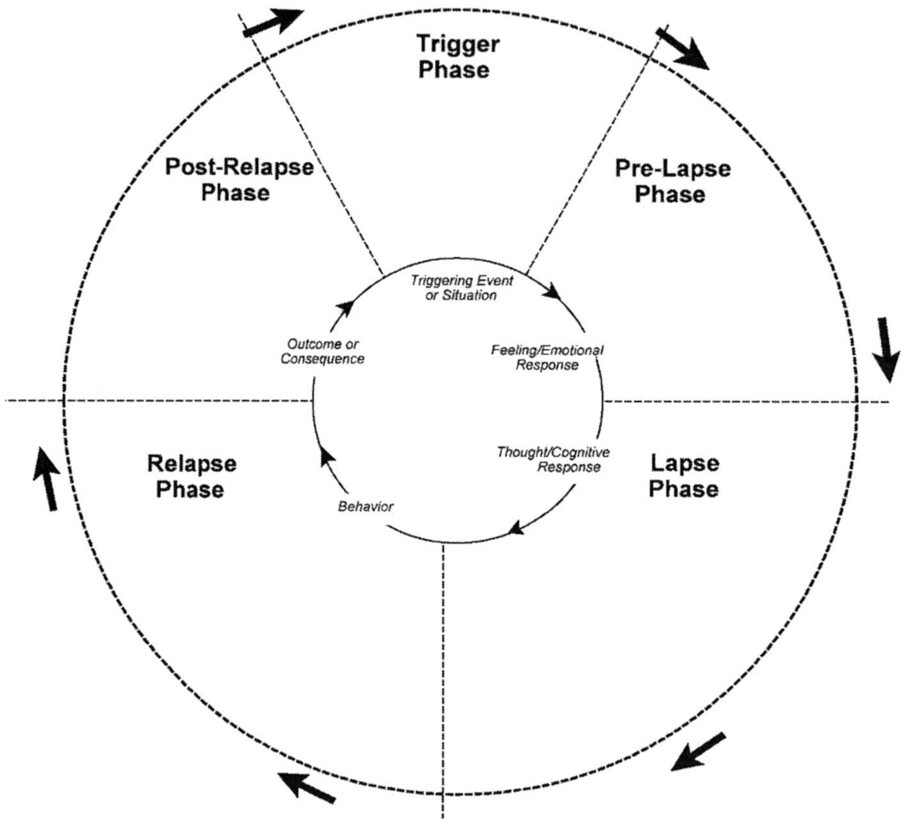

The process of relapse-prevention planning, also long a standing practice in sexual offender treatment, has reasonably been increasingly scrutinized and subjected to much criticism, and rejected by some treatment researchers (for instance, Yates, 2007; Ward, Polaschek, & Beech, 2006). Nevertheless, the model is viable, and particularly when the relapse-prevention plan is visualized as a behavioral safety plan and merely a means to operationalize, or put into actual application, ideas about how to escape from or interrupt dysfunctional behavioral cycles before they lead to dysfunctional behavior – or a "relapse."

After struggling with whether to continue using ideas about relapse and the use of "relapse" terms in developing models of safety planning, we have clearly elected to continue to use these terms and this model as a straightforward, relevant, accurate description of what happens when individuals slip back into and engage in predictable, undesirable, and usually pathological behaviors.

Using the Stages Workbooks in Different Treatment Venues

It is difficult to create a one-size-fits-all workbook for every potential treatment population. The same is true in terms of treatment venue – that is, the location in which treatment is provided, typically some variant of an inpatient or a community- based treatment environment. In turn, the treatment environment to a great degree also reflects some variant of the living environment – residential care, the family home, foster care, group home, etc.

The *Stages of Accomplishment Workbooks* are designed to work with sexually abusive youth in any treatment environment although, as noted, they are likely to have the greatest utility and reach in the residential treatment environment where it is possible to provide a wide, multifaceted, and often intense form of treatment. However, the workbooks are also designed for youths receiving treatment in the community-based treatment environment. Differences in the two treatment settings must be recognized in the use of the workbooks.

Accordingly, workbook use and assignments must be planned and implemented in a manner that best fits the treatment and living environments in which they are applied, and the treatment and management resources available.

Client Motivation

No matter how good the workbook, absent of client motivation all workbooks lack any real or deep utility. Consequently, an early element of treatment involves fostering and nurturing motivation in the client. Fostering motivation is a task for the clinician, unless the client is already motivated. But it is clear that unless the client is internally motivated (rather than by threat of some kind, such as incarceration) it is unlikely that any workbook, no matter how clever, relevant, or well designed, can provide on its own that level of motivation.

For many youths entering treatment for sexually abusive behavior, motivation is key to treatment gain and often needs to be developed through the relationship with the clinician. How to help induce motivation in clients is beyond the scope of this *Clinician's Guide*. However, the topic has been extensively described in the literature (see, for instance, Arkowitz, Westra, Miller, & Rollnick, 2008; Wilbourne & Levensky, 2006).

This concern reminds us again that workbook use is enveloped within the larger treatment environment, and represents an ***element*** of treatment and is, by itself, not treatment, per se. Like education in general, psychoeducation works best when openly and voluntarily received by an enthusiastic learner.

The Therapeutic Relationship

As we discuss the effective use of workbooks in light of client motivation and, in turn, client motivation in light of the therapeutic relationship, it is worth reminding the reader about the therapeutic working alliance, as it is from within this alliance that client motivation is most likely to peak, and client participation is likely to be the greatest. In effective workbook use, and especially for self-learning outside treatment sessions, this alliance is essential, and has been described extensively in the literature (for instance, Bordin, 1976; Castonguay & Beutler, 2006; Hubble, Duncan, & Miller, 1999; Lambert, 1992; Lambert & Bergin, 1993; Norcross, 2002).

Hence, we refer to the idea that all forms of therapy take place within the context of the therapeutic relationship, and that this relationship and working alliance can be characterized in terms of the emotional bonds of the therapeutic relationship, treatment goals shared by both clinician and client, and the agreed upon tasks of treatment. This idea can easily be extended to the clinical assignment and client use of workbooks. Workbooks are most likely to be effective, and most effectively used, not only when embedded within a larger treatment model but within a supportive therapeutic relationship. Without attempting to instruct clinicians in how to form a strong treatment relationship, some of the pertinent elements are reflected in the ten pointers for effective workbook use listed in Section II above. When the clinician recognizes these elements and builds them into work with individual clients, the relationship itself is likely to enhance, support, and make more effective all treatment – including the use and value of workbook assignments.

Pacing Treatment: Twelve Steps

The need to sequence and pace treatment serves as an element in the design and order of the four *Stages of Accomplishment Workbooks*.

The *Stage 1 Workbook* outlines a very simple 12-step model of treatment that describes to youths the pacing of treatment, or its sequence, timing, and elements. In part, pacing means that not everything can be worked on in treatment at the same moment, and also refers to the treatment tasks of the moment. Pacing also means that some things are built upon others, and many treatment issues and concepts can be addressed and learned only after earlier foundation issues and content has been addressed and mastered.

It's worth drawing attention to that simple 12-step model here in order to highlight that the *Stages* workbooks are paced so that their use and their value in treatment moves from the elementary to the more specific and sophisticated over time, based on the acquisition and comprehension, and ideally the application, of earlier learning. Like all treatment, the use of the workbooks is based on the very first step of a 12-step model, before which treatment "proper" cannot effectively begin: the client recognizes that there is a problem that must be overcome, and that he or she is unable to deal effectively with his problem without help.

Briefly, these twelve steps, spelled out for youths in the *Stage 1 Workbook*, provide an excellent illustration of the pacing of treatment, and to a great degree the order and content of the four workbooks and the emotional and cognitive growth and awareness we hope to facilitate in the youths with whom we work. However, it's important to note that, although clearly based on the 12-step model developed and used by Alcoholics Anonymous, a "step" model is neither proposed for use with sexually abusive youth nor used; its only role here is to describe the tasks, steps, and pacing of treatment.

Step 1. Overcoming denial and recognizing and acknowledging a problem.
Step 2 Recognizing the need for help.
Step 3. Accepting help.
Step 4. Becoming honest with one's own self.
Step 5. Becoming honest with others.
Step 6. Willing to change.
Step 7. Ready to change.
Step 8. Ready to explore the damage caused to others.
Step 9. Willing to make restitution in the spirit of healing others and self.
Step 10. Able to accept personal flaws and fully accept responsibility.
Step 11. Building a life based on meaningful relationships, awareness of others, and self- awareness.
Step 12. Living a changed life.

Of course, this is a hopeful sequence, and many youths do not accomplish all of these noble tasks, at least while they are with us in treatment. Nevertheless, many youths do move through these steps, although sometimes in a ragtag way, even if they do not accomplish them all. In recognizing the need to pace, we have not only designed workbooks that pace and sequence tasks from the simpler to the more complex, but we must often also customize and individualize workbooks and treatment in general, to match, follow, and guide the learning curve of each individual client.

Section IV: The *Stages of Accomplishment Workbooks*

Description and Overview

Each of the four inter-related *Stages* workbooks builds upon the previous one, that is, earlier workbooks provide the foundation for subsequent books, in terms of length, depth, and complexity, as well as specific content.

In terms of appearance and use, the workbooks are designed to be user-friendly. Bearing in mind that the workbooks are designed for youths of average intelligence, they are written to be easily understood and in plain language that speaks directly to youth. In addition, and of importance, the workbooks are enlivened with clip artwork and illustrations that make for a friendly visual environment, set a lighter emotional tone, and in a very simple manner bring ideas to life.

Each workbook follows a similar format, and each begins with the same introductory section. Obviously, for clinicians and youths using all of these workbooks, the introduction need not be read and discussed for each subsequent workbook. However, the introduction is important, and should be discussed with clients at least once, and perhaps more if necessary as additional workbooks are brought into use.

As a series, the workbooks move from more elementary material to more complex, more sophisticated, and richer content, and increase in length. The *Stage 1 Workbook: An Introduction to Treatment*, is thus easier to handle, easier to understand and complete, and potentially far less overwhelming and imposing than the *Stage 4 Workbook: Hitting the Target: Making Permanent Change*, which, aside from anything else, has both more pages and more chapters. This arrangement reflects the likelihood that clients will be less put off by workbooks that are briefer in size and contain simpler material, allowing clients to feel less intimidated by voluminous workbook size as they begin their work.

In addition, as the workbooks increase in size, they also increase in their depth of content. They thus allow for a level of gradated success as clients move from one workbook to the next, mastering material in small chunks that provide the basis for both tackling more complex material and feeling successful, confident, and capable as they take on more work.

Each of the four workbooks is aimed at a different aspect of treatment, beginning with orienting clients to treatment. Each provides material and workbook exercises relevant to the development and deepening of treatment that is being addressed in that workbook. Beyond differences in content, the general construction of each workbook is very similar and the same elements of design and use are included in each workbook. In addition to the text, each workbook contains several common teaching elements, each of which are briefly described below.

Teaching and Learning Elements in the *Stages Workbooks*

Key Concepts are included throughout each chapter, summarizing and briefly describing terms and ideas discussed in their relevant sections. Key Concepts thus both teach and remind clients of what they're learning with respect to the definition of important ideas. There are 156 Key Concepts throughout the *Stages* workbooks, which in a few cases are repeated in different workbooks as relevant. Appendix C of the Clinician's Guide contains an alphabetized list of all of the Key Concepts and their definitions.

Thinking Points, like Key Concepts, are also scattered throughout each chapter, providing opportunities for youths to think further about and reflect upon what they're reading, and pose simple questions to themselves. Thinking Points do not require any written work, but are of great importance because they represent key questions for clinicians to ask of clients at any given point in workbook use, and suggest junctures at which to engage clients in a dialogue about their thoughts, emotions, and decisions. Thinking Points additionally provide clinicians with a means for exploring whether and how deeply clients are thinking about and understanding the workbooks and engaging in self-reflection appropriate to their particular cognitive and developmental level.

Written Exercises. All chapters have specific writing exercises for youths to complete, most of which are embedded within relevant text or found at the end of discrete sections. In addition to reading the review section completed by each youth at the end of each chapter, clinicians should also read these written exercises, to ensure that clients understand them and have tried their best to answer them appropriately in terms of both the depth and significance of answers, and in order to answer any questions the youth may have and/or pick up on and further discuss the answers and concepts in terms of clinical interaction.

These written exercises offer great insight into how well youths are comprehending material and how they are approaching their work in terms of motivation and interest. Rather than simply being exercises to be completed, they thus provide the basis for clinical interaction, and even intervention, at several different levels. They can be used by the clinician to explain, to re-direct, and to process and deepen understanding.

What Have You Learned? Review Questions and Learning Exercises. Each chapter concludes with a review section, which amounts to both an extension of learning and a test for comprehension and retention, with material based entirely on the content of the chapter to which the review section is attached. Although it is possible to further test youths for retention and understanding upon completion of each workbook, these review sections are designed to do just that upon completion of each chapter and prior to moving to the next chapter or workbook. In most cases, the items test for conceptual understanding and there are no "correct" answers, per se, as in the case of multiple choice questions for instance.

Accordingly, no "key" is provided by which clinicians may "score" answers, thus it is equally important that clinicians themselves understand the content of the workbooks so that they may judge, or evaluate, how well youths have completed the review questions. It is up to each individual clinician, or treatment program, to decide whether a youth has "passed" the review testing at the end of each chapter, or whether the youth should repeat the review.

Because we want to support learning and retention, the workbooks are designed to allow youths to refer to each chapter and its contents as they complete the review section, and in this case youths are not "cheating" by referring back to the relevant chapter. However, it is again up to the individual clinician or treatment program to decide how to incorporate chapter review testing into their use of the *Stages* workbooks.

Staff Review. The final section to each chapter allows for the clinician and other relevant members of the treatment team involved in the assignment and review of workbook material to "sign off" on the completion of each chapter.

The Use of Written Exercises

Written exercises in the Stages workbooks are not intended to provide answers for youths. They are, instead, designed to aid and develop the skills of self-reflection, exploration, and expression, and help youths think about their own lives and behaviors, and their relationships with others. Clearly, exercises push clients in particular directions regarding the content and goals of the workbooks, and the treatment of sexually abusive behavior in general, but the goal is nonetheless self- discovery, reflection, and expression.

Even though each workbook follows a similar design, some workbooks, and some chapters, include far more written exercises than others. The *Stage 1 Workbook*, for instance, is "light" on exercises and focuses more on ***providing*** information and orienting youths to treatment than having youths complete written exercises (nevertheless, like all of the workbooks, each chapter in this first workbook concludes with a series of questions to be answered, that both tests for retention and provides opportunities for learning).

Conversely, the *Stage 3 Workbook* is focused on understanding and applying the dysfunctional behavioral cycle model. It provides less information and more written exercises, each of which is designed to teach, apply, and reinforce ideas related directly to the dysfunctional behavioral cycle, as well as test for comprehension of the model and the phases of a dysfunctional cycle.

Becoming Familiar with the Workbook Exercises

Written exercises in the Stages workbooks are embedded and incorporated into the text and are spread throughout the four workbooks. The exercises are self-explanatory and require little description in terms of either their purpose or use as the text leading to or following the exercises makes clear the use and purpose of each exercise. The single best approach for the clinician is to review and become familiar with each workbook, the workbook series as a whole, and thus the exercises within them.

Understanding, Assigning, and Applying Exercises .

In many ways, although clinicians may choose to assign particular exercises, it is more likely that clinicians will instead assign whole chapters or perhaps sections of chapters, in which case the process of assigning exercises is taken care of. However, there are different types of exercises, which we will describe in just a moment, and some clinicians may select certain exercises independently of the chapter or text within which they are found. Nevertheless, assigning exercises as "stand alone" assignments is not recommended without having ***first*** used the exercises as designed – that is, as part of a chapter, or at least the section within which any particular exercise is located.

We encourage clinicians to assign exercises as "stand alone," only when they have previously been completed and are being *re*-assigned for any number of reasons. They may have been poorly or inadequately completed the first time around or poorly understood, or they may have been well done and well understood at the time of initial completion, but at a later point in treatment are worth re-visiting and completing again, perhaps from a more sophisticated perspective.

Re-visiting and re-assigning exercises for any number of reasons is a recommended practice. It keeps the workbooks alive, it helps to increase both comprehension and retention, and it ensures the workbooks are not simply static things that disappear into the past as the journey proceeds, like a small town vanishing into history as you speed ahead on a your way across country.

The Reassignment of Written Exercises

For any number off reasons, youths have to be able to repeat written exercises and clinicians have to be able to re-assign them, as well as re-assigning learning reviews at the end of each chapter. However, such re-assignment and re-use will almost certainly involve making a photocopy of the material. Without having this option, it is impossible for clinicians and youths to use these materials in the best possible manner.

Clinicians must take note that all material in these workbooks is copyrighted, which legally prohibits the copying or distribution of any material. Nevertheless, in order to allow clinicians to re-assign and re-visit workbook material, the author and publisher grant permission for the copying and re-use of specific exercises and review sections as needed ***for the sole use of the youth to whom the workbook is assigned***. Under this specific situation, and for this purpose only, the clinician is granted the legal right to make a copy of a specific exercise or review section for a specific client. One option may be for the clinician to keep an extra "clean" copy of a workbook from which an additional copy of a specific exercise or review section may be made when necessary for a particular client.

In being flexible around copyright limitations, in return we ask you to respect our copyright and thank you for modeling attention to legal considerations for your clients.

Types of Exercises

As described, all of the workbook exercises are embedded within the text, but they vary in content, type and format., and content. Many exercises are in the form of "close ended" questions, some of which provide multiple choice answers or a checklist format that allow multiple items to be checked off. Other similar exercises pose "open-ended" questions, such as "How did you feel when ...?" and require a written narrative response.

Other exercises are completely open ended, and induce self-reflection by providing only a "sentence stem" that the youth must complete, such as "When I think of my victim, I ..." In some cases, the exercise is composed of a series of related, but different, sentence stems, and sometimes the youth is asked to complete the same sentence stem several times, hopefully with different answers each time.

Other exercises require the youth to provide a definition, or describe a concept in his (or her) own words. Some exercises ask the youth to describe aspects of his behavior or thoughts or, if in a checklist format, to check off all relevant items. Still others ask the youth to rank items, such as typical emotional responses, types of coping behaviors most frequently used, or the most (or least) supportive relationships in his life, and then follow up with a question or two that has the youth reflect on the answers just given (or items checked off).

Finally, some exercises follow brief stories, or vignettes, that provide examples or illustrate ideas discussed in the text. In these cases, the questions are based on the story, testing for and building the youth's understanding of the story and its point. In some cases the questions are also aimed at building perspective or self-exploration (or both), depending on the story itself. Some of these stories are very brief (a sentence or two), and some a little longer. Sometimes one question follows the story, and sometimes several. In some cases, the workbook re-visits the same story later in the chapter, asking additional questions.

In one form or another, written exercises always pose some sort of question to be answered by the youth, becoming part of the youth's work and journey as the answers are documented directly in the workbook. However, the point of the exercises and their format and placement, how and where in the text they are placed, vary from exercise to exercise. Further, different types of questions aim at different responses, use different types of learning, and have different types of objectives. Some aim at testing knowledge, some at building understanding and retention by repetition, some at comprehension and fostering a deeper comprehension, some at self-reflection, and some at perspective-taking and metacognition.

Using the Thinking Points

Just as different workbooks and different chapters within workbooks use written exercises differently, so too are are Thinking Points are used in different ways in different chapters. These are, in effect, "mind exercises" based on a short series of questions that are posed for the youth to consider, and potentially for the clinician to explore further with the youth. These Thinking Points appear at points throughout the text and in each chapter, and are directly related to the text immediately leading up their insertion point.

Thinking Points are dotted throughout most chapters (but not all), boxed off from the text, and designed to, among other things, challenge and provoke thinking, stimulate self-reflection and self-appraisal, and help youths "locate" themselves in their response to the treatment process at any given time, and additionally, and of great importance, serve as jumping off points for clinical discussion.

Just as clinicians must be familiar with the entire workbook, clinicians should be aware of the various Thinking Points, using and building on them in therapy sessions, and even spinning off additional "homework" assignments as appropriate.

Becoming Familiar with and Using the Review Section

Each chapter concludes with a review section that amounts to a test of knowledge, "What Have You Learned?" These sections are based entirely on material and content relevant to that particular chapter, and vary in the number of questions asked of the youth and the type and format of the questions; they often also include brief vignettes as the basis for one or more questions.

Although the review sections always fit with the content of the associated chapter, they may not "fit" with the youth's developmental or cognitive level, psychological functioning, learning style, or special needs. Some youths will lack the cognitive capacity to fully comprehend questions, the executive capacity to pay attention and complete the work, or the learning skills required to complete written questions. In addition, the youth may feel overwhelmed or intimidated by the review section, and simply give up. Unless you are sure that there is a fit between the work and the client, using any part of the workbooks, and perhaps the review sections in particular, may be ***counter***-productive.

Accordingly, clinicians must be familiar with both the review sections ***and*** the youths to whom the workbooks are assigned. Further, true for the workbooks overall, the clinician may customize and individualize the workbooks whenever necessary or appropriate, and find ways to help youths experience success in workbook completion, including the completion of the review sections.

The Accomplishments of the Youth: Workbook Completion and Treatment Success

With the completion of each workbook, youths are able to show themselves, their families, relevant treatment staff and providers, and others that they are learning about important aspects of their treatment. If the workbook material is being assimilated into their daily lives, they will be able to show people through their behavioral changes that they are able to make changes and apply these new ideas and skills in their everyday lives.

However, the accomplishment of workbook completion, and especially the completion of increasing stages of accomplishment as each workbook is, in turn, completed, must be balanced against larger treatment gains. Without wanting to dampen enthusiasm or minimize accomplishment, we also must bear in mind that workbook completion by itself does not equal "success" in treatment, although it may be a central element.

Section V: Detailed Overview of the *Stages of Accomplishment Workbooks*

This section of the Clinician's Guide provides a more detailed overview of the *Stages* workbooks. Although providing a glimpse into content, structure, sequence, and inter-connectivity, an overview can never substitute for a detailed familiarity with the actual workbooks themselves.

Accordingly, although this overview will provide you with a detailed look at the workbooks, book by book and chapter by chapter, your best and most effective means for becoming familiar with the *Stages of Accomplishment* series is through your careful review of the actual workbooks.

To provide the most thorough overview, each workbook is briefly described as a whole, and then described by chapter, starting with the key points and major headings in each chapter, followed by a general description of the contents and focus of the chapter.

The Youth's Introduction to the Workbooks

Each of the workbooks has essentially the same introductory section. This content highlights and explains that youths to whom these workbooks are assigned are in treatment because of their sexually abusive or sexually inappropriate behavior, that each workbook is part of a set of four workbooks which youths may be assigned throughout the course of their treatment, and that together these workbooks will help youths learn important ideas taught and discussed in treatment. These ideas can help them learn about themselves, their behaviors and attitudes, how their behavior has affected other people, and how to change.

The workbook introductory section also explains that, although not everything in the workbooks is directly about sexually abusive or sexually troubled behavior, each workbook is aimed at helping youths to understand their sexually troubled behavior, leave such behavior in their past, and move into a future that's safer and, hopefully, happier for them and for others.

Youths learn that much of the work involves developing a clearer understanding of themselves and their behavior, as well as the behavior and needs of other people. However, the Introduction also reminds youths that much of the work ***is*** directly about sexually abusive or sexually inappropriate behavior, and that is why they are in treatment at this time. Although honesty and participation often comes only with time in treatment, the development of personal motivation, and the development of a solid therapy relationship, youths are reminded here that if they aren't able to be honest about themselves in their treatment, then it will be difficult for them to meaningfully complete the work in any of the workbooks.

Stage I Workbook: Introduction To Treatment

This first workbook aims to help youths understand and engage in the treatment process, while recognizing that for some youths this is a very new experience. It covers ideas basic to both the treatment of sexually abusive and sexually inappropriate behavior and ideas about treatment itself, at the individual, group, and family level.

The *Stage 1 Workbook* has no written exercises. It more heavily focuses on providing information and orienting youths to treatment than having them complete exercises as they learn. Like all of the workbooks, the *Stage 1 Workbook* has Thinking Points and Key Concepts spread throughout its chapters. Although the focus is on information-giving in this first and shortest workbook, there are as many as 35 questions in the review sections that follow each chapter, and some of these queries have sub-questions within them, all of which test for retention and provide opportunities for learning.

Chapter 1. Introduction to Treatment.

- Major Topics/Section Headings:
- Why Are You in Treatment?
- You're Not Alone
- Goals of Treatment
- Juvenile Sexual Offending
- The Legal System and Treatment
- Sexual Offender Registries
- Honesty, Responsibility, and Denial
- Getting Help

The focus of this chapter addresses the primary reason that youths are in treatment – their engagement in some form of sexually abusive or sexually inappropriate behavior – as well as goals of treatment. The entire workbook, and particularly this chapter, provides more discussion than exercises, and aims at orientation and an early level of engagement in and responsiveness to the treatment process. It discusses labeling issues related to juvenile sexual offending, including the label of "juvenile sexual offender," as well as a brief overview of the legal process and sexual offender registries.

Issues and matters related to the legal process vary broadly by state, province, county, locality, or other jurisdiction that governs or defines them, as well as by the legal charges facing the youth currently or in the near future. Even then legal processes evolve and change over time, such as with changes in state and federal level sexual offender registry laws and compliance regulations. In many cases, youths in treatment for sexual behaviors have not been legally charged and have thus been diverted from the juvenile and adult justice system. Accordingly, this situation offers a perfect example of how information provided and discussed in a workbook must be individualized to best fit the individual client and his or her circumstances.

The chapter also approaches the idea of partnership in treatment, and the roles of honesty, responsibility, and denial in treatment. The Key Concepts section sets the pace for and describes important ideas and terms related to sexually abusive behavior and the work of treatment, and the Thinking Points in the chapter set the tone for the youth to consider what his investment and engagement in treatment might be, as well as his level of honesty and responsibility. Overall, the chapter is both brief and moves slowly. It is aiming at putting a toe in the water to test out its temperature and then come on in, rather than the instant immersion of jumping in at the deep end of the pool.

Aimed at orientation and information-*giving* more than information *getting*, still the 16 questions in the review section require the youth's engagement and test for acquired information and comprehension; a brief story is the basis for several review questions.

Chapter 2. Participating in Your Treatment

- Major Topics/Section Headings:
- Participating in Treatment and Personal Change
- The Treatment Team
- Confidentiality
- Legal Consequences
- Being Honest
- Working with Your Therapist
- The Therapeutic Relationship
- Individual Therapy
- How to Use Individual Therapy
- Group Therapy
- How to Use Group Treatment
- Family Therapy
- Treatment Goals
- The Primary Goals of Your Treatment
- Assessment of Risk
- Changing, and Twelve Steps in Treatment
- Simple Treatment Rules to Live By
- Five Behaviors to Avoid
- Five Rules to Live By

This chapter focuses directly on treatment and how to engage more effectively in treatment. Continuing to provide an orientation, it describes aspects of treatment, including personal participation, the nature and role of the treatment team, and confidentiality and its limitations. The chapter also addresses particular elements of treatment, including: the therapeutic relationship; individual, group, and family therapy; goals and aspirations of each form of treatment; and simple guidelines for effective participation in these modes of treatment. In addition to treatment, the chapter also introduces youths to risk assessment processes, which for many youths, treatment referral sources, and jurisdictional agencies is a significant element in both treatment and life *after* treatment.

Key Concepts in this chapter provide definitions of terms and ideas related to sexually abusive behavior and its treatment, and continue to build an understanding in the youth of treatment-related ideas and constructs. Thinking Points help the youth understand the treatment process and its elements, as well as his or her location in the treatment process at that point.

As with Cchapter 1, and the entire workbook series, you may need to customize the information or its application because many of these elements vary from one youth to another, and depend on the type, intensity, and location of treatment. For instance, there may not be a treatment team, other than the clinician, or the team may be diffuse rather than highly integrated. Similarly, despite a description of group therapy and its role and process, in the outpatient setting group therapy may look very different from its counterpart in residential treatment, if group therapy is provided at all (we certainly hope it is, as it is a central and important element in any form of adolescent treatment). The same is true for family therapy which should be a central feature of all treatment with sexually abusive behavior when a family is available for therapy, but nevertheless may not always be an aspect of treatment. Further, matters pertaining to confidentiality may vary widely among different clinicians, programs, treatment environments, and related circumstances. For these reasons, the clinician must be familiar with workbook material and make adjustments or provide clarifying explanations whenever needed.

This chapter provides information and an overview, using the 35 questions in the review section, rather than the chapter itself, to test for engagement, comprehension, and retention. Review section questions focus more on developing an understanding of treatment, and again use brief stories, or vignettes, as both illustrations and launching points for questions.

As described, the chapter discusses forms of treatment, and describes how youths may effectively participate in different treatment modes, what these treatment modes can offer, and what the youth may gain. As shown in the "Major Topics/Section Headings," Cchapter 2 also spells out a number of "rules" and guidelines for youths to learn and absorb. Each of these sets of thumbnail rules, sometimes known as "heuristics," can aid aid a youth'ss understanding and of how to best engage in treatment, and may be of use to the clinician alsoas well, in helping the youth to effectively engage in treatment.

The twelve basic goals of treatment are listed below, and the clinician is advised to review the other sets of heuristics in this chapter (Twelve Steps in Treatment, 10 Guidelines for Individual Therapy, 12 Rules for Group Therapy, Five Behaviors to Avoid, and Five Rules to Live By). For some youths this may be a lot to absorb, but as the broader content of the *Stage One Wworkbook* is limited, these heuristics represent a central element in learning, and may serve as a focal point in clinical work if necessary.

For the twelve steps of treatment, listed in abbreviated form in Section III of the *Clinician's Guide*, we have previously noted that the only purpose of this heuristic is to describe the tasks, steps, and pacing of treatment. We reiterate: a 12-step model for the treatment of sexually abusive and sexually inappropriate behavior is not used at any other point in the workbooks, nor proposed as a treatment model.

Twelve Basic Treatment Goals

1. Accept responsibility for all of your choices and your behavior, without minimizing or justifying those behaviors, or blaming someone else for your behavior.
2. Be honest about the things you've done, including your sexually abusive and inappropriate behavior.
3. Identify your feelings, thoughts, and behaviors that contribute to sexual abuse and sexually inappropriate behavior, and interrupt (or prevent) them in yourself before they cause harm.
4. Understand the impact of your own history on the way you feel, think, and behave.
5. Understand and choose healthy and appropriate sexual behavior and relationships instead of sexual behaviors that make victims out of other people or yourself.
6. Identify, control, and prevent deviant (unhealthy and inappropriate) sexual arousal and sexual fantasy.
7. Learn to use safe, healthy, and effective coping skills and social skills to deal with issues, concerns, and the challenges of daily life.
8. Develop and show awareness, sensitivity, and concern for others.
9. Build appropriate and healthy relationships.
10. Keep an awareness of sexually abusive and sexually inappropriate behaviors in your daily life.
11. Develop an awareness of risky situations that might cause you to engage in future sexual abusive or sexually inappropriate behavior.
12. Develop and use a safe behavior plan or relapse prevention plan (a plan that helps you to never engage in sexually abusive or sexually inappropriate behavior again).

Chapter 3. Understanding Sexually Abusive Behavior

- Major Topics/Section Headings:
- What is a Sexual Offense?
- Hands-On Offenses
- Hands-Off Offenses
- What Is Sexually Inappropriate Behavior?
- The Elements of Sexual Abuse
- The Three Main Elements of Sexually Abusive Behavior

This chapter is relatively brief and wraps up the *Stage 1 Workbook*. It focuses entirely on further developing an understanding of sexually abusive and sexually inappropriate behaviors; provides definitions, descriptions and discussions of types of sexually abusive behavior, including "hands off" and "hands on" sexually abusive behaviors; and outlines the dynamics of sexually abusive behavior. In particular, sexually abusive behavior is discussed in terms of three classic elements of such behavior: lack of consent, lack of equality, and presence of coercion.

The Key Concepts of this chapter build an understanding and provide further definition of these behaviors, and the review section questions (there are no Thinking Points in this chapter, although the clinician can easily add Thinking Points of her or his own) directly address the youth's understanding of sexually abusive and sexually inappropriate behavior, including asking about the youth's own sexually troubled behaviors.

Stage 2 Workbook: Understanding Yourself

The *Stage 2 Workbook* is aimed squarely at introducing youths to themselves and to the world of interrelated thoughts, emotions, and behaviors. Youths can discover and identify their own internal world and its effects on their external behaviors. There is little focus on sexual behaviors in this workbook, until they are addressed in Cchapter 3 as values and beliefs rather than actual behavior. This workbook emphasizes the relationship between the internal processes of thoughts and feelings and the enactment and externalization of these as attitudes, social interactions, and behaviors.

Chapter 1. Learning About Yourself

- Major Topics/Section Headings:
- Being in Treatment
- Strengths and Limitations
- Fear and Worry Can Hold You Back
- Getting Help and Support

This short chapter begins with the message that "being in treatment isn't just about the things you've done. It's about who you are and who you want to become." The chapter focuses on helping youths to think about who they are, including their strengths and their goals, and what prevents them from setting and meeting their own goals.

Building on the *Stage 1 Workbook,* this chapter first asks youths to reflect upon why they're in treatment and, further, why they're completing the *Stage 2 Workbook,* and whether or not they even believe they need help and support. Youths are guided to think about and clarify their goals in and expectations of treatment, and what they hope to accomplish. Several exercises help youth think about treatment and subsequently describe both their strengths and their weaknesses, including any limitations on their capacity to succeed.

The *Stages Wworkbooks* are neither intended nor designed to address the impact and effect of earlier adverse experiences, which are common among sexually abusive and other troubled youth. In several places, however, the workbooks touch on the outcomes of childhood experiences or trauma. The workbooks may thus serve as important links for clinicians as they recognize the presence and effect of these prior experiences and, at the right juncture in treatment, work on these very important issues with the youth they affect. This chapter briefly touches on processes related to earlier negative experiences, specifically those that create fear and anxiety and/or serve as obstacles to the formation of healthy relationships and trust in others, including those who wish to offer and provide help.

The chapter moves on to address the value of help and support and how to seek such assistance and build a support network. The chapter's short review section focuses on strengths, vulnerabilities, goals, support, and network building.

Chapter 2. Feelings, Thoughts, and Behaviors

- Major Topics/Section Headings:
- Understanding Feelings, Emotions, and Moods
- Understanding Thoughts
- Thoughts and Ideas
- "Rational" Thinking and Thinking Errors
- Understanding Behavior
- Destructive Behaviors: Physical, Emotional, and Mental Harm to Others
- Self-Destructive and Self-Defeating Behaviors
- Dysfunctional Behaviors
- Managing Feelings, Thoughts, and Behavior

As the chapter title makes clear, this chapter explains and explores feelings, emotions, moods, rational and irrational thinking processes, and introduces the concept of thinking errors (addressed in more detail in Cchapter 5). The present chapter also focuses heavily on behaviors, and particularly those that are self-defeating, self-destructive, and/or harmful to others.

Harmful behaviors are also described both in terms of their physical and emotional consequences to others, and in terms of dysfunctional behaviors in general, laying the groundwork for the content of the *Stage 3 Workbook*, which specifically addresses both dysfunctional behavioral cycles and the development of safe behavior and relapse prevention plans.

Chapter 2 concludes by discussing and exploring how youths may recognize and manage their thoughts, feelings, and behaviors, specifically addressing the need to tolerate and contain difficult emotional feelings, so that they don't get "acted out" in antisocial externalized ways or self-harming internalizing behaviors. Introducing the concepts of impulses and urges, the chapter concludes by identifying the need to develop coping skills, further addressed in Cchapter 3 of the workbook.

The review section begins by having the youth define a series of concepts related to the chapter contents, with the focus on ensuring the development of a vocabulary that can aid the youth to recognize and conceptualize important ideas. The review questions also include questions based on stories described in the review section, and test for the youth's understanding of concepts related to thoughts, feelings, and behaviors and their inter-relationship.

Chapter 3. Understanding and Managing Feelings

- Major Topics/Section Headings:
- Using Our Feelings
- Recognizing and Identifying Feelings
- Tolerating Feelings and Managing Feelings and Behavior
- Dealing with Difficult Feelings
- The Importance of Understanding Feelings
- A List of Feelings: Descriptions
- Learning About Your Feelings
- Ranking Your Feelings
- Coping
- Healthy and Unhealthy Coping

This chapter builds entirely upon the ideas and work of Cchapters 1 and 2, helping youths to recognize the value and positive use of their feelings, but also the need to first recognize, identify, tolerate and cope with difficult emotions. This chapter introduces an extensive list of feelings, and asks the youth to first attempt to understand and explain each feeling and then to explore their own feelings, especially those that they most commonly experience.

Coping or dealing with feelings is addressed in some detail, including ideas about "healthy" and "unhealthy coping" (stressing that only *healthy* coping is effective).

Chapter 4. Attitudes, Beliefs, and Values

Major Topics/Section Headings:
Attitudes
Beliefs
Values
What Type of Person Are You?
Keeping Us Safe: Beliefs and Behaviors
Sexual Attitudes and Beliefs

Shifting attention from emotions and their management, this chapter builds upon thought processes and, in particular, attitudes, belief systems, and value clarification. The focus is on how the youth thinks, experiences and expresses attitudes about self and others, his (or her) systems of belief and specific beliefs, what he (or she) values, and whether his (or her) behaviors honor or damage those values and beliefs. The chapter asks the youth to think about how he sees himself.

The review section incorporates several different question formats, including a series of short stories that serve as the basis for many of the questions. This review section contains 36 questions, many of which have several parts to them. As the youth gets further into the workbooks, review sections deepen and amplify the learning process in general, in some cases become increasingly complex as they progress from earlier chapters and workbooks.

Chapter 5. Thinking Errors

- Major Topics/Section Headings:
- Errors in Thinking
- The Way You Think: Your Thinking Errors
- Type 1 Thinking Errors: Unwilling to Accept Responsibility
- Type 2 Thinking Errors: Self-Defeating
- Type 3 Thinking Errors: Narcissism
- Your Most Common Thinking Errors
- Internalizing Thinking Errors and "Scripts"
- Thinking Errors Lead to Thinking Errors
- Three Stages of Thinking Errors

This chapter fully introduces the concept of thinking errors (or cognitive distortions). It builds on the linked ideas that thinking errors: (i) allow people to not take responsibility for their behaviors, (ii) are self-defeating, and (iii) focus people's attention onto themselves, without thinking about other people.

The chapter presents a specific thinking-errors model which breaks thinking errors into three types that have wide-ranging effects, allowing both behaviors that are harmful to others and behaviors that are harmful to self, as well as significantly damaging the client's capacity to socially interact with others in an effective manner. Each category, or class, of thinking errors contains a series of commonly used thinking errors or cognitive distortions, and are specifically with respect to this particular model. The three types of thinking errors are listed immediately below, and the model is detailed in Appendix D, including the thinking errors included in each "type."

Type 1 Thinking Errors: Unwilling to Accept Responsibility.
Type 2 Thinking Errors: Self-Defeating.
Type 3 Thinking Errors: Narcissism.

The chapter contains a number of specific exercises that help the youth focus on understanding and describing thinking errors, including his own commonly experienced thinking errors, and the idea that thinking errors result in internalized "scripts" that people automatically follow, without conscious thought. The goal here is to bring these automatic thoughts and unconscious scripts into conscious awareness, so that change can be considered and made – the process often known as cognitive restructuring. These sections of the chapter use simple stories to illustrate the ideas and offer a way for the youth to both consider his own patterns of thinking and develop the capacity for perspective taking, an important precursor to the development and experience of empathy.

The chapter concludes by going beyond thinking errors to the three stages of thinking errors, and specifically relating these to engagement in sexually abusive behavior:

Stage I. Pre-Abuse Cognitive Distortions: "Contributing and Leading"
Stage II. In-Abuse Cognitive Distortions: "Allowing and Supporting"
Stage III. Post-Abuse Cognitive Distortions: "Justifying and Strengthening"

A more detailed description and illustration of this model is provided in Appendix E.

Stage 3 Workbook: Understanding Dysfunctional Behavior

This workbook returns the youth to work directly related to sexually abusive behavior. Workbook 3 is used to work entirely on developing and applying an understanding of behavioral cycles, and help youths to recognize and understand their own dysfunctional and problem behaviors. The last chapter in the workbook points youths towards the development and creation of safe behavior/relapse prevention plans which are closely related to behavioral patterns that, like all patterns, are both repetitive and predictable.

Keep in mind that, although workbooks can be used in stand-alone fashion, they are designed with a clear sequence in mind and intended to be used in this sequence. In this case, the *Stage 3 Workbook* continues to build upon the ideas about behaviors and thinking errors that were described and worked on in the *Stage 2 Workbook*.

Chapter 1. Dysfunctional Behavioral Cycles

- Major Topics/Section Headings:
- Managing Behavior
- What Affects Behavior?
- The Behavioral Cycle
- The Sequence of the Dysfunctional Behavioral Cycle
- The Parts of the Dysfunctional Behavioral Cycle
- Dysfunctional Behavioral Cycles as High Risk
- Interrupting the Cycle

This chapter lays the foundation for the workbook by first describing behavior management and the influences on behavior that surround youths and are also often internally present in terms of their thinking and emotions. Concepts and ideas about dysfunctional behavior, in particular, are also discussed.

Patterns of behavioral are explained in the form of five basic and inter-related elements, each one of which leads to the next: (i) event/trigger, (ii) feeling (iii) thought, (iv) behavior, and (v) outcome, leading back into the next event, contributing to or potentially starting another behavioral cycle. This simple model is transformed into a behavioral cycle that can easily be illustrated, as shown in Figure 5.

Trigger Event. The behavioral cycle starts with a *situation* or an *event* that serves as a *trigger* to a feeling-thought-behavior sequence.

Feeling/Emotional Response. The event triggers an *emotional response.*

Thoughts and Ideas. The feelings/emotions trigger a *cognitive response*, or thoughts, ideas, beliefs, or attitudes.

Behavior. Thoughts and ideas lead to a *behavior* or *action* of some kind.

Outcomes. All behaviors have *outcomes, results,* and *consequences.*

New Event. Behavioral outcomes feed back into and help shape the next situation or event.

Trigger Event. The new event triggers to a new cycle of *event-feeling-thought-behavior-outcome-event.*

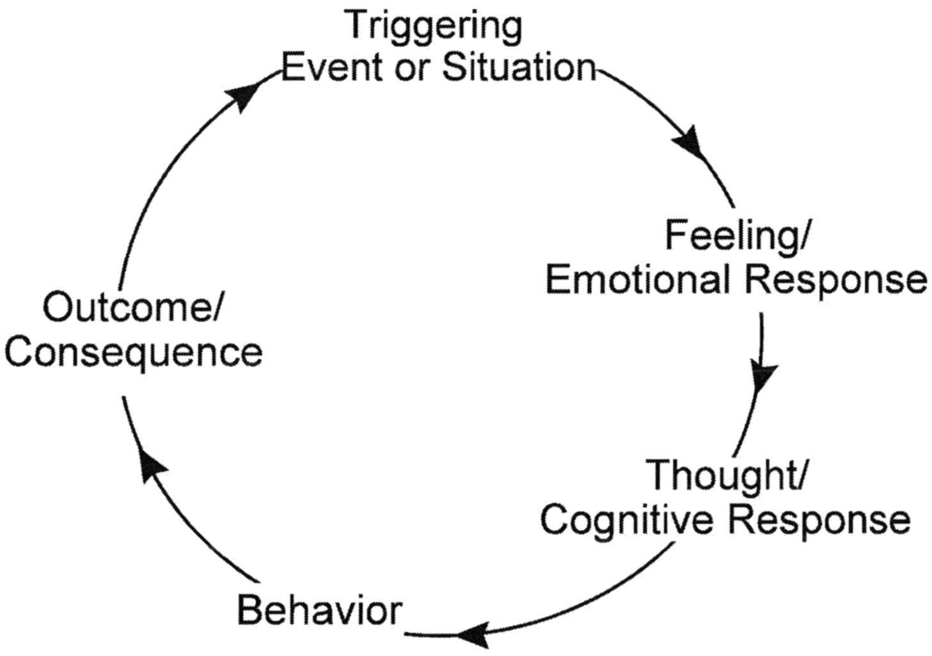

Once introduced, the dysfunctional behavioral cycle is described more fully, first in terms of its parts, as described above and as shown again in a slightly different way (six elements, with the first separated into "event" and "trigger") in Figure 6.

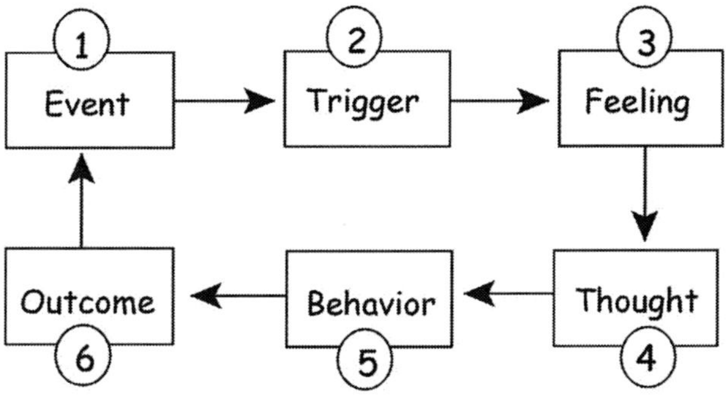

Following the discussion, a written exercise of eight questions asks the youth to apply the ideas of dysfunctional behavior and the dysfunctional behavioral cycle to one recent instance of his (or her) own behavior. The chapter moves on to further discuss and simply illustrate each elements, or "leg," of the dysfunctional cycle, demonstrating how these individual elements incrementally add up to the entire cycle.

This chapter uses several more exercises, combined with Thinking Points and Key Concepts to further develop ideas about dysfunctional behavior and behavioral cycles. The cycle is additionally identified as "high risk," introducing the concept of high-risk factors and situations that are further discussed in Cchapter 3 of this workbook. Also introduced is the idea of "interrupting," or "escaping," the behavioral cycle. The review section for this chapter is relatively short.

Chapter 2. Phases of the Dysfunctional Behavioral Cycle

- Major Topics/Section Headings:
- Phases of the High-Risk Cycle and "Relapse"
- Understanding Each Phase
- Phase 1: The Trigger Phase – Getting Set Off
- Phase 2: The Pre-Lapse Phase – Building Up
- Phase 3: The Lapse Phase – Planning
- Phase 4: The Relapse Phase – Acting Out
- Phase 5: The Post-Relapse Phase –After the Acting Out
- Putting the Phases Together

This lengthy chapter teaches a particular model, and all of its exercises are aimed at drilling home and applying these ideas. The model itself is not complex, but, as shown in Section III, has several linked elements that add up to the whole. This chapter takes this model, breaks it into its component parts and explores each part, and then assembles the parts into the whole model. Because of the chapter's length, the detail of its content, and the amount of writing required by the exercises and the review section, this chapter is not only exhaustive but may potentially exhaust the youth as well. So ... take the demands of the chapter into account when assigning it.

The chapter first introduces and describes the concepts of relapse and phases, and subsequently reviews and explains each of the five phases built into the model, first by separating and "explording" each phase, as shown in Figure 7.

Phase 1: The Trigger Phase – Getting Set Off.
Phase 2: The Pre-Lapse Phase – Building Up.
Phase 3: The Lapse Phase – Planning.
Phase 4: The Relapse Phase – Acting Out.
Phase 5: The Post-Relapse Phase – After the Acting Out.

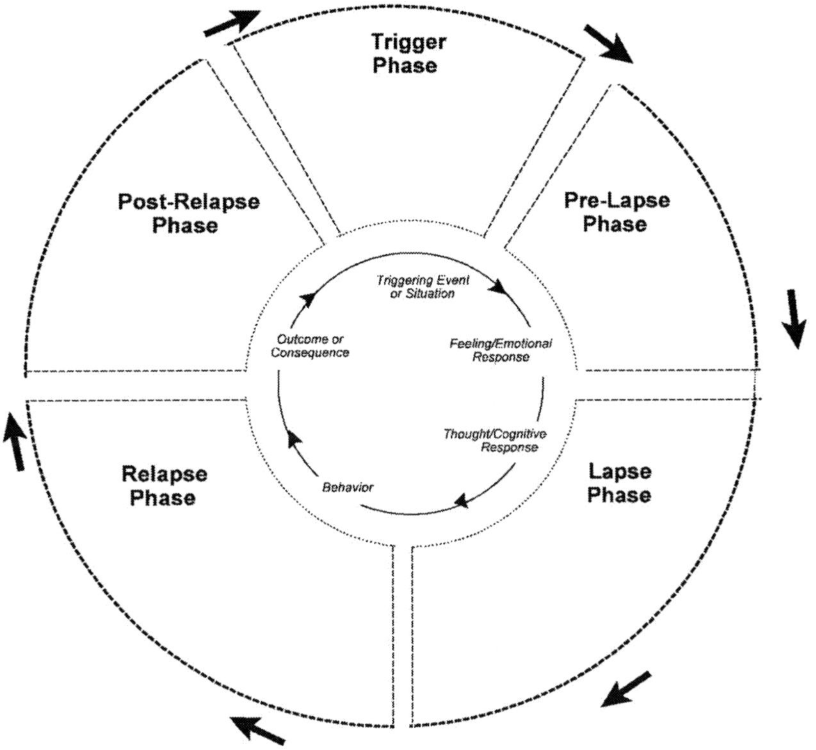

After exploring and working through the individual phases, the chapter re-assembles the phases into the complete phased cycle shown in Figure 8, which now includes a more detailed description of the elements that are embedded within each phase of the cycle.

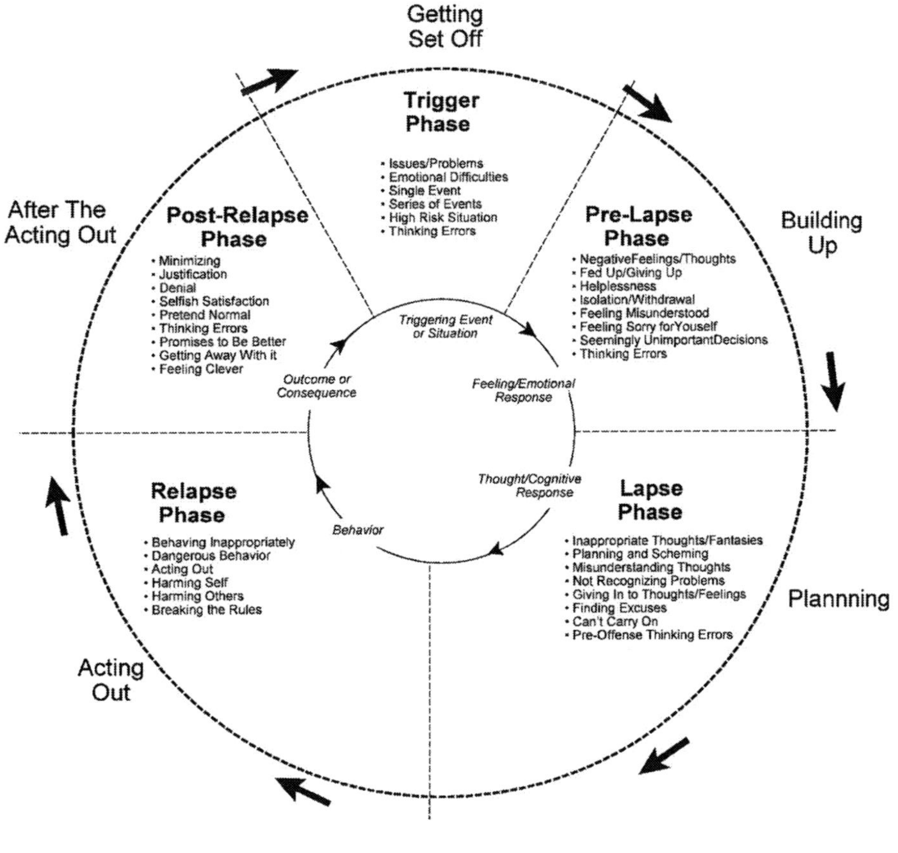

The chapter's extensive review section includes illustrative vignettes designed to help the client apply the ideas.

Chapter 3. High-Risk Situations and Behaviors

- Major Topics/Section Headings:
- Urges and Cravings
- Triggers, Dangerous Situations, High-Risk Situations, and High-Risk Factors
- The Elements of Risk
- Seemingly Unimportant Decisions
- Denial and Minimization
- High Risk and Decision-Making Skills
- Keeping Secrets
- Protective Factors

Beginning almost immediately with a brief illustrative story to explain, explore, and develop perspective taking, Cchapter 3 describes and provides examples of high-risk situations and factors. Moving on to describe urges and cravings (introduced in the *Stage 2 Workbook*), Cchapter 3 flags these experiences as high-risk warnings, and again uses a vignette to illustrate and further explore the concepts.

Building further, the chapter returns to triggering events, and ties them to dangerous situations, high-risk situations, and high-risk factors. These elements are related to repetitive patterns of dysfunctional behaviors, and because they are commonly taught in sex abuse-specific treatment, it is important for youths in treatment to learn and explore these ideas as they may be exposed to them in other treatment programs and venues. In discussing the elements of risk, thinking errors and attitudes and beliefs that support antisocial behavior are flagged as high-risk factors in the perpetration of sexually abusive and sexually inappropriate behavior. Likewise, urges and cravings that cannot be tolerated and managed are shown to play a role in risk factors, aggravated by the Problem of Immediate Gratification ("pig"), as it is sometimes called.

The chapter thus addresses ***internal*** risk factors, such as antisocial attitudes and beliefs, and ***external*** risk factors, such as entering or remaining in situations or being with people that engender or encourage (even unintentionally) either self-destructive behavior or behavior that is harmful to others. The chapter also identities the major concept of seemingly unimportant decisions (SUDs), as links in a chain that can lead to both antisocial behavior in general and sexual recidivism in particular.

Both through discussion and a writing exercise, denial and minimization are addressed in the chapter, including the many variants and subtleties of denial. This concept is followed by the role and nature of decision-making skills in recognizing and dealing with elements of risk. The chapter provides a simple model for decision-making, focusing on the elements of: (i) responsibility in decision-making, (ii) thoughtfulness versus impulsiveness, and (iii) the long-term effects and outcomes of the decision-making process.

Chapter 3 not only covers risk factors and elements of risk, but also introduces and addresses protective factors: "It's not all about risk. It's also about protection *from* risk. You not only face risk in your life, and high-risk situations, but you also have strengths that can help protect you from making mistakes and getting into high-risk situations."

The chapter explains and describes these protective factors, and helps the youth to explore the protective factors, people, organizations, and other resources in his (her) life.

The review section is relatively short for this chapter, but the chapter itself involves a number of exercises, making this another writing heavy chapter. By the end of Cchapter 3, as youths approach the final chapter and the completion of the *Stage 3 Workbook*, they have a come a long way from the *Stage 1 Workbook*.

Chapter 4. Behavior Management, Staying Safe, and Preventing Relapse

- Major Topics/Section Headings:
- Elements of a Behavior-Management Plan
- Behavior-Management Planning
- Relapse-Prevention Planning
- Steps in Relapse Prevention
- The Re-offense Chain and High-Risk (Dangerous) Situations
- Breaking the Re-Offense Chain
- Your Relapse-Prevention Plan
- Coping with Feelings and Thoughts
- The Benefits of Escaping Dysfunctional Behavior and Avoiding Relapse
- Getting Help
- Strengths and Goals
- Developing and Using Your Relapse-Prevention Plan

The final chapter in the *Stage 3 Workbook* helps youths to understand and develop means and plans for preventing future behavioral problems, and especially behaviors that are destructive to themselves and others, including a recurrence of sexually abusive behavior (i.e., relapse).

The chapter describes the similarities and differences between behavior-management plans and relapse-prevention plans: the behavior plan is more general, and the relapse-prevention plan aims at preventing a recurrence of dangerous behaviors. The chapter explores the ideas and elements of such plans, the rationale for safety planning, and the difference between ***making*** safety plans and actually ***using*** them. As experienced treatment professionals know, some variant of safety or relapse-prevention planning is basic to the treatment of juvenile sexually abusive behavior, yet many relapse-prevention plans are either poorly developed or simply go unused, for any number of reasons.

Much of the chapter re-visits and builds upon the ideas of Cchapters 1, 2, and 3, and tests for retention and comprehension of these ideas through written exercises, as well as self-evaluation. Exercises urge the youth, at this point in his treatment, to honestly appraise his prior sexually abusive or sexually inappropriate behavior, although like many of the exercises found throughout the workbooks, allow for an "I'm not ready to discuss this" answer.

Asking youths questions can create genuine discomfort or anxiety for the youth. Asking him to acknowledge and describe in writing his sexually abusive behaviors may understandably cause the youth concern. The decision made by the youth about how to answer a question like this should not be taken as the most profound reflection on his (or her) treatment, as there may be many surrounding contextual complications and factors that affect the decision-making process. Nevertheless, the youth's choice to answer or not answer a question like this may certainly offer some insight into how far he or she has come in treatment to this point.

The remainder of the chapter provides for the actual development of a relapse prevention plan, and includes many of the elements previously addressed in the *Stages* workbooks. The relapse prevention process thus incorporates an awareness and the identification of troublesome elements: triggers, seemingly important decisions, cravings, and other warning signs such as deviant sexual fantasies, emotional dysregulation, and thinking errors. As a meaningful and useful learning experience, the plan also recognizes and identifies coping strategies that will be used to help avoid relapse, supportive people and other helping resources, and personal strengths and goals.

The review section is again relatively brief, since so much written work has been completed as part of the chapter itself. The workbook, however, concludes with some "parting words" that extend past the review section and treatment staff review of the material, acknowledging how far the youth has come at this point in treatment, and especially when all three workbooks have been completed thus far.

Stage 4 Workbook: Hitting the Target. Making Permanent Change

Phew! Imagine how your client must be feeling about the work that he's completed so far. There is a genuine reason to offer congratulations to youths who have completed all three prior workbooks and have arrived at the final workbook in the series, and to recognize their accomplishment.

This fourth and final workbook aims at building relationships, establishing social connection, and taking responsibility through making social reparation. It also aims at the recognition and development of relationships that are healthy and satisfy the youth, adding meaning to his or her life and allowing the youth to add meaning to the lives of others and the community-at-large. These issues and topics lie at the heart of sex abuse-specific treatment; more so than psychoeducational concepts, models, and tools, it is the nature and quality of social relationships, social membership, and the social relatedness through which our behavior is anchored, has meaning, and links us to others that can support or restore pro-social behavior.

Addressing these issues is complicated for anyone, and certainly for still-developing adolescents. For youths who have engaged in serious antisocial behavior and are already disconnected in some or many ways, these issues are perhaps even harder to recognize and work through. The topics of this final workbook represent the "top of the hill" climbed by youths in treatment. The material, learning processes, tasks, and content of the first three workbooks have set the pace, built the endurance, and taught the youth how to approach the work and accomplish its goals, and thus develop the level of sophistication and "workbook maturity" that will be of great help in completing this final workbook in the series.

For these reasons, this workbook is designed to be completed only after much groundwork has been laid upon which the Stage 4 work is built and accomplished. The *Stage 4 Workbook* is "high end" in content, with topics that are best tackled by youths "trained" and matured in workbook use and conceptually prepared to recognize its ideas and their importance and thus most meaningfully engage in the work

This workbook uses a considerable number of illustrative vignettes as the basis for many of its writing exercises, which are found in all chapters.

Chapter 1. Thinking About Others: Empathy and Caring

- Major Topics/Section Headings
- Empathy in Action
- Taking Perspective
- Empathy Blocked
- Letting Empathy Guide Your Decisions
- Remorse
- Morality

The chapter addresses relationships from the perspective of the connections allowed by empathic and caring relationships. It begins by describing empathy as "understanding and caring about others," and "feeling connected to others," recognizing that "one key step in the development of empathy is feeling that people understand and care about you!" This maxim sets the tone for a chapter, and indeed the whole workbook, that is about two-way relationships, connections, and communication, and not only what the youth has to do for others. This is an important element in any empathy, relationship, and community building work.

Following several exercises that address caring relationships in the youth's current life, and the youth's own level of caring and concern for others, the chapter introduces perspective-taking, an element that has figured in the design of many exercises in the earlier workbooks. The text describes perspective-taking as a ***cognitive*** process (that is, recognizing someone else's perspective doesn't necessarily require emotional insight). Several stories are provided, each followed by exercises that aim at addressing and building perspective, and thus support the youth's recognizing and taking another person's point of view. Perspective-taking can also be considered a crucial element in the capacity to experience empathy, in which the empathic experience goes beyond cognitive perspective-taking and is experienced on an emotional level.

Building on the vignette exercises, the chapter returns to empathy by having the youth consider what blocks or interrupts, or allows us to "switch off" empathy, and the importance of allowing empathy to guide his (or her) decisions and relationships with others, allowing healthy and pro-social choices and helping connecting the youth to other people.

This content easily leads to a description and discussion of remorse and subsequently moral reasoning, providing exercises in both cases that further these ideas, deepen understanding, and provide opportunities for self-evaluation and self-reflection. The chapter concludes with Thinking Points, Key Concepts, related exercises, and a relatively short review section that continue to build on and reinforce the ideas of the chapter and provide the basis for the following chapter, which addresses victim awareness.

Chapter 2. Victim Awareness and Clarification

- Major Topics/Section Headings
- Physical Harm
- Emotional Harm
- Harm to Families
- Harm to the Community
- Harm to Yourself
- Victim Awareness: Healing the Harm
- Victim Clarification
- Increasing Victim Awareness
- Victim Empathy Essay, Victim Letters, Apology Letters
- Victim Questions
- Your Own Past

Victims and victimization have been addressed in prior workbooks, but this chapter concentrates on sharpening the youth's understanding of victimization and the damage his sexually abusive or sexually inappropriate behavior has caused. It takes an emotional tone, and thus goes beyond cognitive perspective-taking and applies an approach that attempts to have the youth "feel" the effects of his behavior on others.

The goal here is to not to induce shame or highlight irreparable damage, but instead to allow the youth to move toward developing remorse for his behaviors and to recognize that he is able to engage in a reparative and healing process that can help him and his victims to move forward.

The chapter describes physical and emotional harm and the victims of such harm, including the family, the community, and the youth himself, in addition to the direct victim(s) of sexual abuse. A detailed exercise follows that pulls the youth into the discussion. There is a special edge to looking squarely at who the victims are, as in many cases, the victim's family and the family of the offender are one and the same, and the victims of juvenile sexual offenders are often their younger siblings or other younger family members.

The chapter moves to the related subjects of victim awareness and reparation, or healing the harm caused, and this theme predominates in the remainder of the chapter. Discussion and an exercise built around victim awareness is followed by a description of the meaning, purpose, and process of victim clarification. This is the process by which offenders face (or clarify) the full consequences of their sexually abusive behavior and begin the process of making amends of some sort, directly or indirectly, to the victims of their behavior. Amends may include apology letters and eventually – if allowed by the victim and his or her family on the advice of a therapist and with appropriate follow-up – face-to-face therapeutic sessions with their victim(s). Such a meeting is especially pertinent when the victims are family members (usually younger), and thus it becomes a part of family treatment and reunification.

Preparations for victim clarification are discussed and worked on through written exercises. The focus is on increasing victim awareness and helping the youth become more attuned and sensitive to the victim's experience through the use of victim empathy essays, victim letters, and apology letters, examples of which are provided.

A *victim essay* exercise asks the youth to write about his (or her) victim's experience, imagining what the victim may have experienced and may now be feeling. A *victim letter* takes a slightly different approach by having the youth create a fictional letter written to him by the victim, in which the abuser writes from the point of view of the victim. The *apology letter* offers the most direct way for the youth to take responsibility for his sexually abusive or inappropriate behavior. The text stresses that the apology letter is an exercise ***only*** at this point, and may or may not eventually be sent. Under any circumstances, apology letters should ***never*** be sent without the permission of the victim and the victim's family if he or she is a child.

Many young people who engage in sexually abusive behavior have themselves experienced adverse or traumatic childhood experiences, and many have themselves been sexually or physically abused. The chapter concludes with the possibility of the youth's own experience of being victimized at some earlier point. As noted previously in the *Clinician's Guide*, the *Stages Workbooks* are not designed to address the youth's own experiences of abuse, neglect, or other forms of maltreatment, but the clinician must remain aware of this possibility. The final element in the chapter aims at encouraging the youth to recognize and deal with these issues if they are present and at work in his (or her) life, and in that case to understand how his own victimization may have contributed to his victimization of others.

The chapter concludes with a brief review section.

Chapter 3. Community Service

- Major Topics/Section Headings
- Communities are Shared Spaces
- Community Learning and Community Service
- Community Membership
- Your Environment
- Building Community
- Understanding Community Building
- Community Service
- Learning Through Community Service

As the chapter explains, the word "community" comes from a Latin word that means "common, public, shared by all or many." This is the theme for the chapter, building on and moving the workbook from empathy, responsibility, and reparation to a larger sense of social relatedness and attachment. The chapter emphasizes the value and meaning of being connected to and being part of a community, and describes the nature and benefits of community learning, community service, and community membership, and the responsibility that belongs to all of us in helping to create and nurture the community environment in which we live.

The overall theme is the reciprocal and two-way relationship between the youth and his (or her) environment, the role of the community in providing support and nurturance, and the youth's role in helping to either build communities or damage them. The exercises focus on understanding the community process and community membership, and the youth's understanding of his community and his role in that community, as well as his desired goals. Community service and community learning and their relationship to one another are described, with relevant exercises designed to spark exploration of what community service opportunities may be present for the youth, and examine the nature of community service as both reparative and restorative, in addition to building a sense of connection.

As in previous chapters, the review section here is brief, in consideration of the amount of written exercises within the body of the chapter.

Chapter 4. Learning to Communicate

Major Topics/Section Headings
Understanding and Communicating Your Ideas, Feelings, Needs, and Experiences
Obstacles to Communication
Saying What You Mean to Say
Listening to Yourself
Non-Verbal Communication: Speaking Without Words and "Body Language"
Hearing Others: "Active" Listening
Direct Communication: Assertiveness versus Aggression

"I" Statements: Speaking for Yourself
Being Heard and Hearing Others: 15 Rules for Effective and Honest Communication
Giving and Getting Feedback
Rules and Guidelines for Giving and Receiving Feedback
Problems with Communication

Communication as a key skill is emphasized in this chapter, with a focus on building an awareness of communication and the essential skills upon which effective communication is built. Again, illustrative stories are used to bring ideas to life, increase comprehension and meaning, and provide a basis for written exercises. As with relationships in general, communication is also described as a reciprocal and mutual, two-way, process.

This detailed chapter addresses many aspects of communication, including giving and receiving feedback. Early in the chapter, description and exercises are provided that focus on personal communication and obstacles to such communication, as well as basic skills of effective communication:

- The ability to recognize our own feelings, and put those feelings into words.
- The ability to understand someone else's point of view, and recognize their feelings.
- The ability to say the things we want to say in a way so that they get heard.
- How to listen to other people so that we hear the things they're ***really*** trying to say, and not just what we think they're saying ("active listening").

Two exercises in this chapter include interaction with staff and peers. For youths in a residential or group treatment environment, this exercise is easier to complete than for those in community-based treatment, but the tasks associated with the exercise can still be accomplished through interactions with adult care givers such as case workers, probation officers, or teachers, and using school mates, friends, or same-aged family members as peers. The questions in this case are related to communication and not sexually abusive or antisocial behavior, and are thus "safe" and neutral questions, and involve the primary question, "how well do you think I communicate my thoughts and feelings, and how well do you think I listen to others and understand what they mean?"

In addition to communication ***style,*** the chapter also focuses on the ***content*** of communication and learning to say what is intended, and how to say it. These topics are again illustrated by vignettes that allow an objective view of effective and ineffective communication, as well as related exercises that prompt the youth to think about obstacles to effective communication.

Non-verbal communication, including "body language," is discussed, with accompanying vignettes and exercises, as well as a description and the principles of "active" listening – paying close attention to both the words and the non-verbal communication of the other person. Going back to communication style, the difference between "assertiveness" and "aggression" is discussed, as well as the value and use of "I" statements in direct and effective communication.

Before moving to a discussion of feedback, a heuristic of 15 "rules" is provided as an aid to effective communication. These guidelines are useful for anyone, and provide the sorts of pragmatic "rules" for communication and social interaction valuable to youths with autistic-spectrum diagnoses:

1. Establish common ground.
2. Be non-judgmental.
3. Communication is interactive.
4. Be flexible.
5. Face the person you're talking to.
6. Pay attention to what the other person is saying.
7. Don't fidget or be distracted.
8. Pay attention to your non-verbal communication.
9. Pay attention to the other person's non-verbal communication.
10. Remain calm and respectful.
11. Respond, don't "react."
12. Don't interrupt.
13. Finish listening before you begin to speak.
14. Listen carefully for the main idea.
15. Ask questions.

As feedback is important communication skill in treatment and in daily life, the chapter provides a strong focus on definition, description, guidance, and rules of thumb, in both giving and receiving feedback; as usual, the section is followed by exercises that address the youth's understanding of the feedback process. This section offers an excellent example of the difference between workbook knowledge and real-life application. That is, a youth may demonstrate a clear grasp of the ideas and practices of feedback, but in actual application may show little understanding or skill in actually giving or receiving feedback. Hence, workbook learning should never be mistaken for the acquisition of ***applied*** learning or skills, and must thus be tested for and practiced in real life.

The related guidelines are described here in name only, and the clinician should refer to the chapter itself for a detailed description and explanation.

- Six "Golden" Rules of Feedback
- Eight Guidelines for Positive Feedback
- Six Things to Remember in Receiving Feedback
- Receiving Feedback in a Positive and Open Style
- Avoiding a Negative and Closed Style in Receiving Feedback

The chapter concludes with some consideration given to communication problems, followed by a detailed review section that addresses and re-visits many of the ideas described and discussed in the chapter.

Chapter 5. Healthy Relationships

- Major Topics/Section Headings
- Types of Relationships
- The Reality and Difficulty of Friendships
- Understanding Healthy Relationships
- Relationship Problems and Sexually Inappropriate Behavior
- Intimate, Romantic, and Sexual Relationships
- Healthy and Unhealthy Relationships
- Growing Healthy Relationships
- Recognizing Healthy and Unhealthy Relationships
- Recognizing Boundaries
- Recognizing Healthy and Unhealthy Sexual Relationships
- Power and Control in Relationships
- Assessing Your Relationships: Healthy or Unhealthy?
- Barriers to Sexual Re-offense/Continued Sexually Inappropriate Behavior
- Five Behaviors That Define Sexually Abusive Relationships
- Five Simple Rules for Healthy Relationships

Chapter 5 amounts to the final working chapter in this and the Stages workbooks, as the chapter 6 content, described below, primarily provides a wrap-up and reflective overview for the youth. Chapter 5 focuses entirely on relationships, relationship-building, and establishing healthy relationships, as well as understanding healthy sexual relationships and, hence, healthy sexuality.

The chapter begins by discussing and distinguishing between types of relationship, ranging from close to more distant, noting clearly that many youths who experience difficulties in building relationships feel lonely and disconnected from others, including age-peers. These youths want relationships, but often don't know how to build or keep them, and feel awkward and unsure of themselves. This issue is a central one for many of the youths you treat. Understanding relationships and the quality and meaning of these relationships is often key in helping to understand driving forces behind juvenile sexually abusive behavior. In part, the goal here is to help recognize these difficulties, since at least some of the youths who will be using these workbooks struggle with relationships or have given up on them. The acknowledgment provided here will also help these youths recognize that they are not alone in experiencing difficulties in establishing healthy and satisfying relationships.

The chapter helps youths to understand the characteristics of healthy non-sexual and sexual relationships, types of sexual relationships, and links between relationship difficulties and sexually troubled behaviors, and uses vignettes and exercises to develop the ideas further and involve the youth in thinking and exploring more deeply these ideas.

Intimacy in healthy relationships is explored, in terms of closeness and connection more than in terms of sexual intimacy, and healthy relationships are described by several basic elements:

They must be consensual.
They must be appropriate.
They must be free of harm to the people in the relationship.
They must be free of harm to the people outside of the relationship.

Healthy and unhealthy relationships are additionally described in terms of 12 characteristics that distinguish healthy from unhealthy relationships, shown in more detail in Appendix F of the Guide.

1. Respect.
2. Caring.
3. Boundaries.
4. Honesty.
5. Trust.
6. Dependability.
7. Consistency.
8. Openness and Sharing.
9. Investment.
10. Connection.
11. Mutuality.
12. Consent.

Twelve Characteristics of Relationships	
Healthy Relationships	**Unhealthy Relationships**
Respectful. Healthy relationships involve each person respecting the other, and wanting the best for each other.	Disrespectful. There is a lack of respect in unhealthy relationships, in which people may say unkind things to each other, put one another down, or hurt each other's feelings.
Caring. In healthy relationships, both people care for and about each other.	Uncaring. In unhealthy relationships, there is a lack of concern or caring for the other person.
Good Boundaries. People in healthy relationships know how far they can go with the other person and how close to get, and respect what the other person wants and doesn't want in the relationship.	Poor Boundaries. People in unhealthy relationships don't recognize, think of, or care about the boundaries of the other, and may take what they want or step where they're not really welcome.
Honesty. In healthy relationships, people are honest and truthful with each other.	Dishonesty. In unhealthy relationships, there is a lack of honesty and truth.
Trust. People in healthy relationships know that they can trust the other person, and that the other person will not take advantage of them.	Mistrust. There is a lack of trust and openness in unhealthy relationships, and a sense of certainty about the other person.
Dependable. In healthy relationships, people can count on the other person to be there for them and follow through on promises and commitments. People in healthy relationships can rely on one another.	Undependable. One or both people in unhealthy relationships are not dependable. People in unhealthy relationships can't be counted on, and can't rely on one another.
Consistent. Healthy relationships don't change from day-to-day, and neither do the people in them. People in healthy relationships know what to expect from each other.	Inconsistent. Things in unhealthy relationships change and shift quickly, and people in unhealthy relationships don't necessarily know what they can expect from the relationship or each other.
Open and Sharing. People in healthy relationships share their ideas, their thoughts, and their feelings. They not only share their secrets and their experiences, but they also share with one another their skills, their support, and the things they each own.	Closed and Secretive. People in unhealthy relationships aren't open and keep secrets from one another. They hold their thoughts and feelings inside and don't share them with each other.
Invested. People in healthy relationships are invested and interested in one another, and want to hear about the things that others in the relationship think and feel.	Uninvested. In unhealthy relationships, people are not really interested in the thoughts, feelings, and experiences of the other person.
Connected. In healthy relationships, people are connected to one another, and come to learn about and understand each other.	Disconnected. People in unhealthy relationships are not well connected, don't understand each other very well, and often misunderstand one another.
Mutual. In healthy relationships, people share things in common. Things that are good for one person are good for the other.	Selfish. People in unhealthy relationships are less interested in the needs of the other person, and more interested in their own needs.
Consensual. People in healthy relationships both want the relationship.	Non-Consensual. Unhealthy relationships often involve one person forcing the relationship onto the other.

The text describes boundaries in relationships as invisible "fences" that allow people to know where they can and cannot go. This discussion is followed by a description of the role of power and control in relationships, particularly sexually abusive relationships, leading into several exercises that focus on the quality of the youth's own relationships in terms of the characteristics that mark relationships as healthy or unhealthy. These exercises are built around the use of a relationship "graph," two examples of which are shown in Figure 9.

The chapter concludes with the five simple behaviors to avoid and five simple rules to follow that were introduced in Cchapter 2 of the *Stage 1 Workbook*. The two lists are used to characterize and depict five behaviors that mark unhealthy sexual relationships and five behaviors that help maintain healthy relationships. These two related sets of guidelines are, in effect, the converse of one another, although they do involve some changes in wording:

Five Behaviors that Define Sexually Abusive Relationships

1. **Taking something that's not yours.** Sexual offenders use the bodies of other people, and take from them their freedom, privacy, safety, and often their innocence.
2. **Not asking permission.** Sexual offenders don't ask permission for what they take.
3. **Invading space.** Sexual offenders invade the physical, emotional, and sexual space of others.
4. **Keeping secrets.** Sexual offenders keep secrets, and force or require others to keep their secrets as well.
5. **Taking it out on someone else.** Sexual offenders take out their frustrations and get their needs met literally by taking advantage of another person.

Five Simple Rules for Healthy Relationships

1. Don't take things that don't belong to you.
2. Always ask permission.
3. Respect boundaries.
4. Don't keep secrets.
5. Don't take things out on other people.

Chapter 6. Epilogue: Your Final Words

This final brief chapter offers the youth the opportunity to summarize and reflect upon of the work he (or she) has accomplished.

It begins with well-deserved congratulations, recognizing that youths who have completed all four workbooks have worked hard, learned a lot, and are able to understand and think about things in new and different ways.

From these few words on, there are just nine exercises, all in the form of sentence stems or simple statements that are both summative and reflective in design and nature.

About myself, I've learned...
About others, I've learned...
About my role in the world around me, I've learned...
About my behaviors, I've learned...
About my coping skills, I've learned...
Other lessons I've learned...
As I go back out into the world around me, I plan to...
My goals...
My final words in this workbook...

The final chapter of the final workbook ends with the words we hope have been instilled as goals for the youth's future: "Be Safe! Help Others Be Safe!"

Section VI. In Conclusion

Workbook Accomplishment and Treatment Success

Without in any way minimizing the work accomplished by youths in completing these workbooks, we must reiterate that the completion of workbooks alone does not equal "success" in treatment. Neither does it mean, that in their real lives and daily behaviors and interactions youths will be able to live by the skills they've learned though using the workbooks, no matter how great or genuinely meaningful the achievement.

All workbooks, including the *Stages of Accomplishment*, must be used, tied into, and understood as part of the broader treatment environment's ideas, and learning, which is value-tested in that larger environment for acquisition understanding, retention, and application.

Appendixes

Thinking Errors

Thinking errors can fuel both antisocial and self-defeating behaviors, and can be grouped into three types of thinking errors, or "cognitive distortions."

Combined, these thinking errors result in a series of interactive cognitions that include self-defeating, self-destructive, relationally disconnected, and antisocial thoughts, beliefs, and attitudes, that reinforce and generate still more thinking errors.

Type 1 Thinking Errors: Unwilling to Accept Responsibility – *"It's Not My Fault"*

These cognitive distortions allow people to not take responsibility for their behaviors.

- Denial. The youth simply pretends it didn't happen, and might even try to fool him/herself into thinking it didn't happen. If he/she denies it ever happened, maybe it will go away.
- Shifting the Focus. The youth tries to get people's minds and attention onto something else, and distract them from the real issue.
- Blaming Others. The youth blames the problem and his/her own behavior, onto someone or something else.
- Blaming the Victim. The youth blames the victim, as though he/she wasn't at fault, and somehow the victim brought it on him/herself.
- Intellectualization. The youth tries to use ideas and intellect to sidetrack issues and out think the opposition, finding excuses and explanations.
- Innocence/Playing Dumb. The youth simply act as though he/she didn't know it was wrong or against the rules, or pretends he/she didn't know better.
- Rationalization. The youth finds reasons, explanations, and excuses for what he/she did.
- Justification. The youth find reasons to explain the "correctness" of what he/she did, as though it was really okay.
- Minimization. The youth downplays the importance of what happened, or its meaning.
- Dismissal. The youth simply disregards, ignores, or brushes aside what happened or other people's feelings as though they don't matter.
- Angelic Thinking. This is a victim stance, in which the youth portrays him/herself as a wonderful person, incapable of breaking the rules or harming someone.

Type 2 Thinking Errors: Self Defeating – *"I Can't!"*

These thinking errors are self defeating and interfere with personal growth and self esteem.

- Catastrophic Thinking. The youth magnifies the impact of negative experiences to extreme proportions.
- Hopelessness. The youth assumes that nothing will ever work out, and that things will always go wrong.
- Over Generalization. Something goes wrong in one situation, and the youth applies it to all situations.
- Black-and-White Thinking. The youth see things as "all-or-nothing;" things are either one way or the other.
- Oughts, Shoulds, and Musts. The youth feels life ought to be a certain way, or he/she should do something, or things must go the way he/she wants them to.
- Negative Predictions/Fortune Telling. The youth predicts failure in situations yet to happen because things have gone wrong before.
- Projection. The youth makes negative assumptions about the thoughts, intentions, or motives of another person, which are often "projections" of his/her own thoughts and feelings about the situation.
- Mind Reading. The youth feels that others should know how he/she feels or what he/she wants even though he/she doesn't tell them.
- Labeling. The youth labels him/herself or someone else in a negative way, which shapes the way he/she sees him/herself or that other person, often for simplistic reasons.
- Personalization. The youth treats a negative event as a personal reflection or confirmation of his/her own worthlessness.
- Negative Focus. The youth focuses mainly on negative events, memories, or implications while ignoring more neutral or positive information about him/herself or a situation.
- Avoidance. The youth avoids thinking about emotionally difficult subjects because they feel overwhelming or insurmountable.
- Emotional Misreasoning. The youth draws an irrational and incorrect conclusion based on the way he/she feels at that moment.

Type 3 Thinking Errors: Narcissistic – *"Me, Me, Me"*

These cognitive distortions focus the attention of youths onto themselves alone, without thinking about others.

- Life Is Too Hard. The youth feels that life is just too unfair, and somehow owes him/her more.
- Entitled. The youth feels as though he/she deserves good things, even if he/she doesn't have to work for them.
- Victim Stance. The youth feels as though he/she is the victim of the whole world, and that he's the one who's been harmed.
- Grandiose. The youth feels as though he/she is better or more important than other people, or others should and do look up to him/her.
- Revenge. The youth feels as though he's been wronged and is allowed (or entitled) to get his/her revenge.
- Personalizing It. The youth feels as though the rules are applied only to him/her, instead of everyone, and that people and things are against him/her personally.
- One Upsmanship. The youth feels he/she has to do better than everyone else, and show everyone that he/she is the best.

Three Stages of Cognitive Distortions and Sexually Abusive Behavior

Stage I. Pre-Offense Cognitive Distortions: Contributing and Leading

- Critical to the sexual offense are those thinking errors that get things boiling, and contribute and lead to a sexual offense.
- These are the ideas, beliefs, and attitudes that mix thoughts and feelings together, and move the youth towards sexually aggressive behaviors, setting the groundwork for and justifying the movement towards sexually aggressive behavior.

Stage II. In-Offense Cognitive Distortions: Allowing and Supporting

- In most cases, the mind doesn't switch off during the offense itself, with no recognition of right or wrong.
- Thinking errors don't simply occur prior to and after the offense. They are constant, and in effect during the offense. Thinking errors not only drive the offense in the first place, but allow and support the offense while it is occurring.

Stage III. Post-Offense Cognitive Distortions: Justifying and Strengthening

- These are the thinking errors that continue to develop and evolve after the offense.
- In any model where remorse, shame, or some other form of social conscience doesn't kick in to re-shape the offender's experience of the offense, thinking errors only serve to justify the offense, reinforce the behavior, and strengthen the offending behavior and, indeed, the thinking errors themselves.

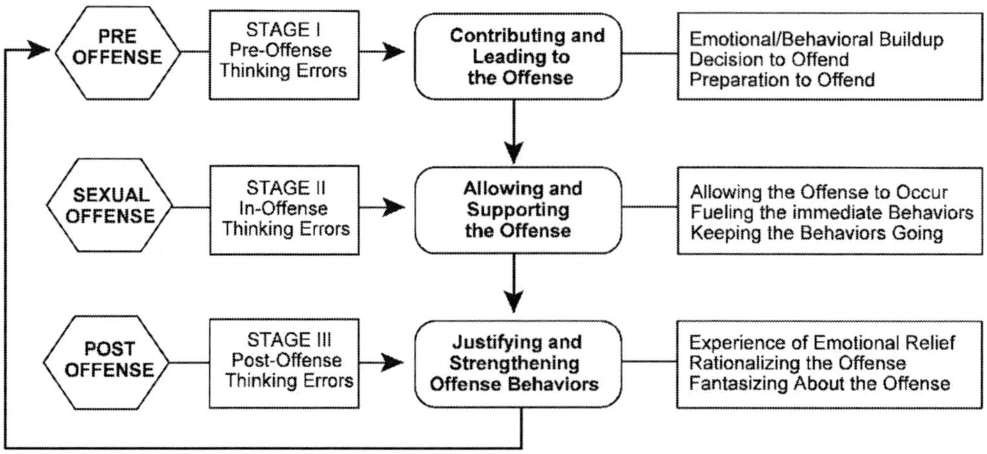

One Safe Step at a Time: Alternative to the Dysfunctional Cycle

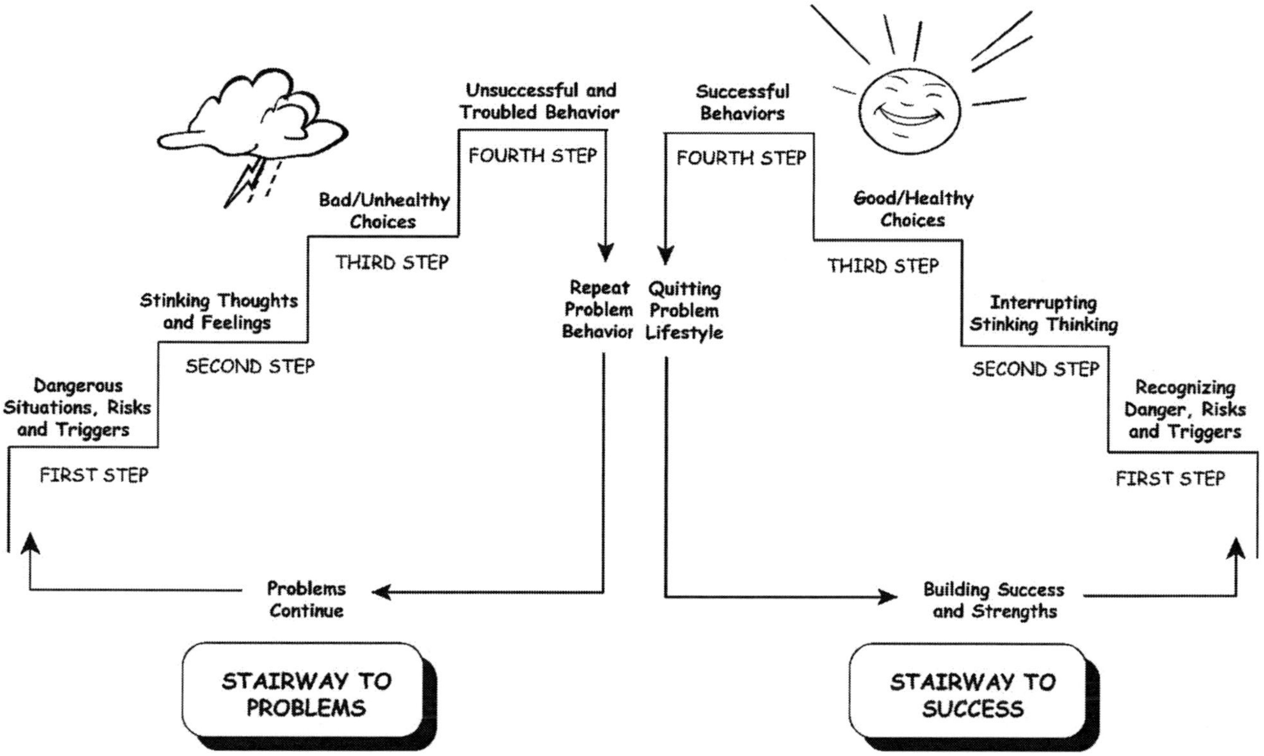

Simplified Dysfunctional Cycle

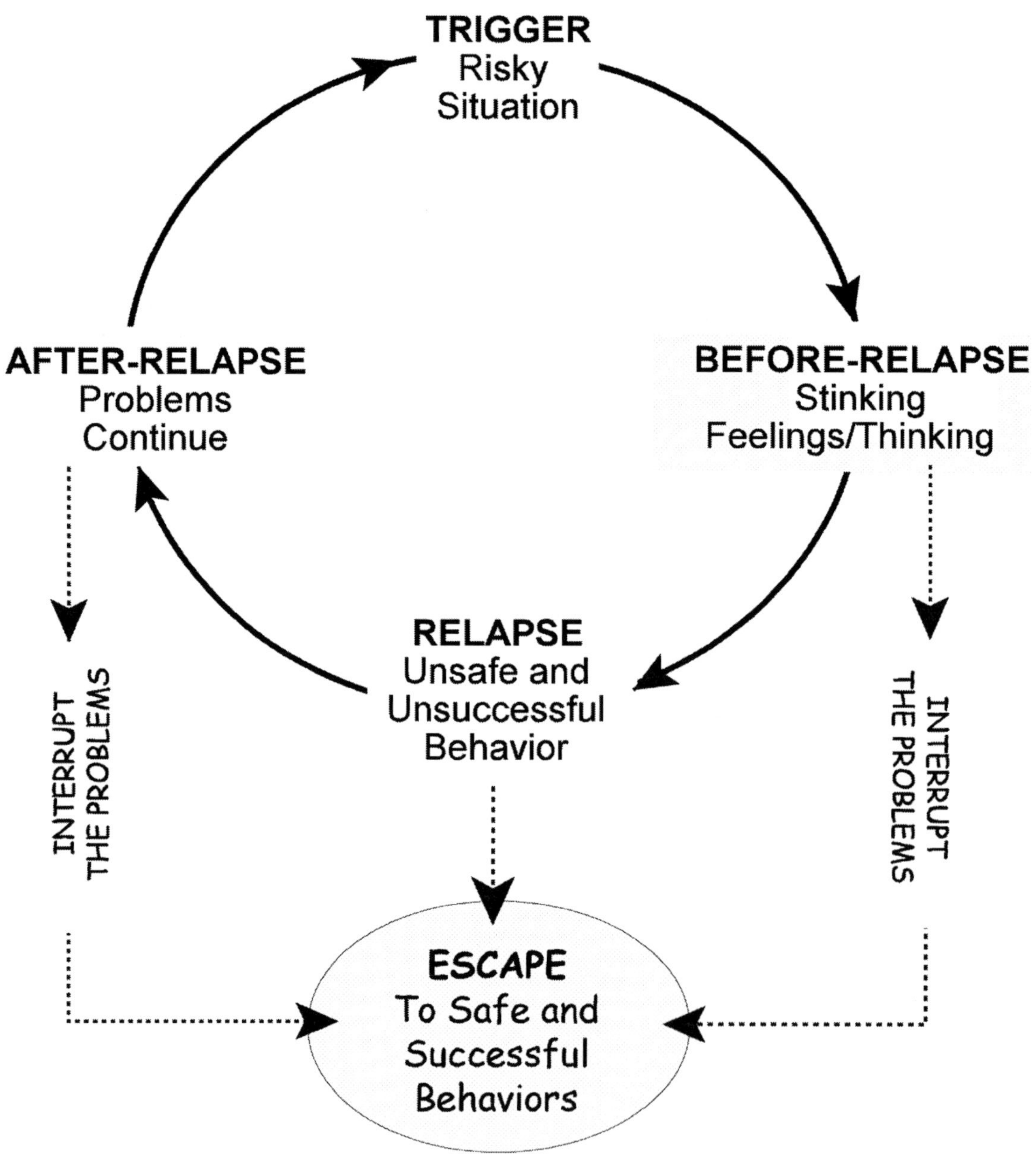

Listing of Key Concept Definitions

1. Acting Out. Turning feelings and thoughts into negative behaviors.
2. Active Listening. Giving undivided and direct attention to someone else when they're talking in a genuine effort to listen to and understand their point of view. Active listening means showing someone that you are listening to them, and interested in what they have to say.
3. Aggression. Acting in a hostile or destructive way, using force or hostility to communicate with others as a way to get them to do what you want. Aggression is a threatening, angry, or demanding type of behavior used to control others. Aggression quite often violates the rights of others.
4. Alliance. The relationship built between two or more people working on the same goals. In treatment, the alliance is built to try to help you make those personal changes described in this workbook.
5. Antisocial. Attitudes, values, behaviors, and interactions with people that are negative, do not help others or yourself, and quite often are destructive and harm others and yourself.
6. Appropriate. Socially acceptable and proper, does not cause harm or lead to problems.
7. Assertiveness. Being confident and self-assured, and speaking your mind clearly. Being assertive means standing up for yourself and your needs, or speaking out for the things you think are important.
8. Assumption. A pre-set point of view taken without knowing the point of view to be correct. When we think we know something to be true without checking the facts, we are making an assumption.
9. Attitude. The way you feel or think about something, your mental outlook, or the position you take and often make clear to others on whether you like or dislike something or somebody.
10. Barrier. An obstacle or device, sometimes for our own protection or the protection of another person, that prevents us from crossing from one point to another, or slows us down.
11. Behavior Management. The things we do to control our behavior so that it doesn't become destructive to us or to others.
12. Behavior. The things we do that can be seen by other people, including our actions, our words, and the way we treat other people.
13. Belief System. A collection of beliefs that affect your attitude and values, and help shape the way you treat other people and live your life.
14. Belief. Something that you think is true or something in which you place your trust.
15. Body Language. A type of non-verbal communication in which physical gestures, postures, and movements convey meaning without the use of words, including facial expressions.
16. Boundary. A limit to where we can go physically and/or emotionally. Boundaries between people involve how close a person wants other people to get, and serve to keep distance between people. The personal territory, or "space," with which people surround themselves in order to keep themselves private or safe. It's different in different cultures and relationships, but in the U.S., it's usually no closer than about 18 inches, or the space inside a hula hoop. Boundaries are not limited to physical space, though. They also apply to people's emotional "comfort" level, involving privacy, for instance, how much people want to share about themselves or what they want to know about someone else, or how friendly one person wants to be with another. Boundaries refer to both physical space and emotional space.
17. Boundary Violation. Stepping into someone else's personal boundaries/space without being invited or welcome.
18. Child Neglect. No actual physical harm is done to a child, but his or her needs are not met by a parent or another person responsible for the child's care. Neglect can include not providing necessary meals, housing, clothing, or medical care, and can also include simply not taking care of children, allowing them to be placed in dangerous situations, or allowing them to see things they shouldn't see, such as family violence, sexual acts, pornography, or drug use.
19. Choices. Decisions to behave in a certain way when faced with different possibilities of what to do.
20. Clarify. To explain or make clear, and to remove uncertainty.
21. Coercion. Getting people to do something you want them to do, even though it may not best for them. Coercion usually involves threats, tricks, bribes, gently forcing others, or in some way getting others to give in to your needs.
22. Cognition. A thought or idea, and the ability to think.
23. Cognitive Distortions. Another way to describe thinking errors, twisted and harmful ideas that do not reflect reality.
24. Communicate. To tell or "express" to others how we feel, what we are thinking, what we need, or the experiences we've had, and letting people know about us. Communicating is a two-way process. It also means joining or connecting with others, by learning about them, and their needs, experiences, feelings, and thoughts.
25. Community. Individuals who share something in common and feel connected through the things they share; people who share a common living space, such as a home, a neighborhood, or a town, or people who share ideas, beliefs, and values.
26. Community Learning. Gaining knowledge about ourselves and others and developing more skills through our involvement and interaction with our community.
27. Community Service. Something that individuals or groups of people do for their community in order to benefit their community in some way; contributing to the community.
28. Confidentiality. Keeping sensitive treatment information private, sometimes between just two people, unless the person in treatment gives permission. Confidentiality can apply to many situations outside of treatment, such as in friendships or business relationships. In treatment, however, confidentiality includes maintaining the privacy of information shared between you and your therapist, as well as information that you or others share in group therapy.

29. Consensual. Voluntary, involving the agreement of all parties without being coerced, manipulated, or forced.
30. Consent. Freely giving someone permission to do something, without being coerced or forced.
31. Consequences. The outcomes, or the products, of the choices and decisions we make and the things we do. Consequences can be good or bad. We want to help you make choices that have positive consequences and not negative ones for you or for other people. The result of behaviors. Consequences are the outcomes of the choices we make and the things we do. Consequences can be good or bad.
32. Cope. Dealing with and managing different situations, difficult feelings, or negative thoughts so that situations, feelings, and thoughts don't overwhelm you. To deal successfully with a problem, without resorting to negative or antisocial behaviors. Someone who is coping can successfully and positively face and deal with responsibilities, problems, or difficulties in a calm manner.
33. Craving. The feeling that people get when they feel they really want or need something.
34. Denial. Pretending that something didn't happen when it did, or making it sound much less important or severe than it really is.
35. Destructive. A force or quality of a behavior or an action that damages and causes harm to things or people, and sometimes destroys things. The condition of harm or injury caused by our behaviors to others or ourselves, including physical, emotional, and mental harm.
36. Deviant. An idea, thought, or behavior that is very different from the things most other people believe or the ways most other people act. Deviant ideas or behaviors can refer to many things, including just doing things differently than others. For this reason, although "deviant" is often considered in a negative light, being "deviant" may also mean simply being "different," or being "yourself." However, "sexual deviancy" involves sexual ideas and behaviors that are outside of the mainstream and are often considered unacceptable, illegal, or harmful to others, such as adult sexual interest in or adult sexual behavior with a child.
37. Deviant Fantasy. A fantasy, daydream, or idea that involves harm to someone else, or that is very different from the way most other people do things.
38. Deviant Sexual Fantasy. A fantasy, daydream, or idea of having a sexual relationship in which someone is harmed or humiliated, or involves sex with younger children or people who aren't as powerful as you, who are unable to make decisions for themselves, or who don't know better.
39. Deviant Sexuality. An unhealthy and inappropriate sexual arousal and sexual fantasy that may involve adult or adolescent sexual arousal to a child or sexual behaviors that are physically or emotionally harmful.
40. Digital Sex. Inserting your fingers into someone's vagina or anus for sexual reasons.
41. Distress. Mental or physical suffering or pain; feeling emotionally troubled.
42. Dysfunctional. The description of our thoughts, beliefs, behaviors, or patterns of doing things when they don't work well, don't lead to effective solutions, are self-defeating, or are destructive to ourselves and/or to others.
43. Dysfunctional Behavior. Actions that don't accomplish anything positive, prevent people from improving their lives, contribute towards difficulties and problems, and are often self-defeating or harmful to other people.
44. Dysfunctional Behavioral Cycle. a series of feelings, thoughts, and behaviors that lead from one problem to another, and lead to the same problems and behaviors being repeated over and over and over again.
45. Elements of Sexually Abusive Behavior. A sexual offense can usually be considered to have occurred when one or more of these three elements are present. (1) Lack of consent, (2) lack of equality, and (3) presence of coercion.
46. Emotions. Another word to describe certain types of feelings.
47. Empathy. The ability to identify with, understand, and care about another person's situation, feelings, or motives. Understanding and caring about the feelings of another person; understanding how another person feels, and experiencing some of those feelings yourself, and because of that wanting to help others who are in distress.
48. Environment. The physical, emotional, and social space we live in and that surrounds us. We not only live in our environment, but are also part of our environment.
49. Equality. When two people are pretty much evenly matched, in terms of age, intelligence, size, and authority.
50. Essential. Absolutely necessary; required and important; something very basic upon which other things are built.
51. Exhibitionism. When someone exposes his or her sexual parts to someone else. This behavior is also sometimes known as "exposure" or "flashing."
52. Experiences. The things that we've been through, done and that have happened to us, and the way that we've been affected by these things in our lives.
53. Exploit. Take advantage of or selfishly use someone else for our own personal gain and without regard for their feelings.
54. Feedback. Communication from others that reflects how we are communicating to others. It involves one person letting another person know how he or she is coming across to others in the way they talk, what they're saying, and the ideas they're presenting. Because communication is two-way, feedback not only means giving this information to others about their communication style, but also getting information from others about our own communication style.
55. Feelings. Our basic responses to our experiences that show how those experiences are affecting us. Our emotions and the way that we're affected by the people, circumstances, and events around us.
56. Fondling (or "molesting"). Touching someone's sexual parts or touching a person in a sexual way, without the person's permission (consent) or against the person's wishes.
57. Frottage. Purposely rubbing up against someone for your own sexual pleasure, usually when fully clothed, and sometimes when the other person doesn't even know that you're purposely rubbing against him or her.
58. Genuine. Related to honesty, not pretending to be something you're not, and that you really are the person you present yourself to be. It means being sincere, and not trying to trick or manipulate other people.

59. Goals. The targets we set for ourselves, and the sorts of things we want to achieve in our lives.
60. Healthy. Well and free of physical, emotional, or mental illness; contributing to good condition and well-being; leading to good outcomes.
61. Help. Assistance that people give, or offer to give, that can make things better for others. Things that people do (or offer to do) to make the situation better, lend a hand, offer support, and assist people who are in trouble to get to a better and safer place.
62. Honesty. Telling the truth, being trusted by others, keeping your word, and being genuine.
63. Ideas. Beliefs and opinions about things, or plans to turn thoughts into actions (or behaviors). Ideas include our thoughts, and the things we think about other people and the world around you.
64. Identity. The view or image that people have about themselves and who they are and what they can do. The things and ideas with which people associate or the people to whom they feel connected.
65. Impulse Control. Sometimes also known as "urge control," this involves the ability to not give in to an urge, an impulse, or a craving.
66. Impulse. Similar to an "urge," in which you act without thinking or act on an urge.
67. Impulsive. To act without thinking, to act on an urge.
68. Interaction. The connection (or engagement) between two (or more) people and the effects that each has upon the other in relationships and communication.
69. Internalization. The process of becoming so used to thinking or acting in a particular way that it becomes part of the way you automatically think and do things, and becomes part of your set of beliefs about the way things are or should be.
70. Internalize. The process of accepting an idea, attitude, or belief into the way you think, or learning ideas, beliefs, values, and attitudes that are incorporated within yourself and become part of the way you think.
71. Interrupting the Cycle. Stopping the cycle from progressing to a more negative phase. This is sometimes called "breaking" the cycle. The ability to recognize a dysfunctional behavioral cycle, and stop the cycle from developing further or getting worse.
72. Intimate. Feeling very close and connected to one another, sharing a special relationship that is usually quite private.
73. Irrational Thinking. Thinking that is not clear, that is not based on accurate information or ideas, and that leads to poorly thought-through decisions and behaviors. Irrational thinking does not lead to sensible thinking.
74. Judgmental. Forming opinions about other people, and judging them as good or bad in some way.
75. Justify. To explain why something happened or why something was the right thing to do, also often to excuse behavior and make it seem right, when it actually wasn't.
76. Lapse. An error in judgment, a slip in thinking during which thinking returns to former ideas that may be inappropriate or negative.
77. Limitations. Similar to vulnerabilities, the qualities that weaken our abilities to accomplish our goals and to make things better.
78. Manage. To stay on top of and appropriately control something, or to be in charge of something.
79. Manipulate. Trying to control other people and trick them in some way into doing something that you want them to do, usually for your own advantage or for personal gain.
80. Mindset. A collection or set of attitudes, beliefs, and values that together define the way people feel and think about the world, affects their behavior, and shapes their expectations and relationships with others.
81. Minimization. Making something seem much smaller or less significant than it really is; pretending that something is no big deal, when it actually is a big deal.
82. Moods. Usually a collection or "color" of a set of emotions. Moods affect the way we feel about ourselves, others, and the world around us. They sometimes affect the ways we interact with others.
83. Morality. Understanding the difference between right and wrong, and thinking and behaving in a way that supports and helps other people.
84. Myth. A belief shared by a number of people that something is true when it really isn't true.
85. Narcissism. An attitude and sense of self that is marked by self-preoccupation, a sense of being more important than others, and a lack of empathy.
86. Needs. Something we are lacking, or those things that help us to feel better, deal better with the world, or allow us to better take care of ourselves and our responsibilities.
87. Non-Consensual. Things you do without the clear permission of the other person. Even if the other person gives consent, the sexual act is considered non-consensual if the other person is not old enough or not capable of giving real consent (or permission).
88. Non-verbal communication. The use of facial expressions, tone or volume of voice, physical posture (the way you hold your body), and interactions with others to convey meaning, without the use of spoken language. Non-verbal communication includes smiling and frowning, head nodding and head shaking, and paying attention to or ignoring someone while talking or listening to them.
89. Obligation. Something that is required or expected of us, such as following through on promises, taking care of people who depend on us, and being honest and trustworthy.
90. Obstacle. A barrier that gets in our way, and prevents us from meeting our goals. Obstacles are things we have to remove or overcome for us to proceed further.
91. Oral Sex. Sexual acts involving the mouth or tongue, such as licking the penis, vagina, or anus.
92. Overcome. To struggle successfully against a difficulty or disadvantage. We overcome things when we work through situations that hold us back. We overcome disadvantages by challenging our own limitations, defeating the things that stand in our way, and then meeting our goals, anyway.
93. Overwhelmed. To feel overcome, overpowered, or crushed by something such as a feeling or thought.

94. Penetration. A sexual act that involves pushing the penis, fingers, or an object into the vagina or anus. Oral sex may also be considered "penetration" if it involves putting your tongue into someone's vagina or anus, and similarly putting your penis into someone's mouth may be considered to be penetration. However, acts of penetration usually refer to placing the penis, fingers, or other objects into someone's vagina or anus.
95. Perpetrator. Someone who commits an offense against another person or commits a crime, such as someone who sexually abuses someone (although the crime can also be a robbery or a physical assault, for example).
96. Personal Changes. Alterations that take place within you, and especially in the ways that you feel and think about yourself and other people, your beliefs and attitudes, and the things that are important to you. Positive personal change means that you are better able to feel happy with yourself, form good relationships with other people, and live a productive, satisfying, and safe life.
97. Personal Strengths. Positive qualities that help us to achieve goals and get things done. Strengths help us to improve on a current situation, and they help us to keep our lives in good shape.
98. Perspective. A way of seeing things and making sense of a situation, an attitude that shapes the way we see the world, our point of view. Seeing the world through someone else's eyes.
99. Phase. A temporary period of time during which feelings, thoughts, and behaviors develop, progress, and change.
100. Plan. A method for getting something done. We use a plan to accomplish a goal.
101. Platonic. Relationships that involve friendship and not romantic or sexual behavior.
102. Pretend Normal. Acting as though everything is okay, even though things aren't okay at all.
103. Pro-social. Attitudes, values, behaviors, and interactions with people that are positive and support people and social expectations and rules.
104. Problem of Immediate Gratification. Gratification means getting your needs met. The Problem of Immediate Gratification – or PIG – means that some people feel they have to get their needs met right away, regardless of who might be hurt in the process, and this leads to many problems for them and for other people.
105. Processing. Thinking about and understanding our feelings and our experiences.
106. Protective Factor. Something that decreases the possibly harmful effects of a risk factor. Something that helps to keep someone safe from risk.
107. Rape. The act of forcing someone to have sexual intercourse, involving penetration of the vagina or anus.
108. Rational Thinking. Thinking that is based on reasoning, or taking care to think through and sense a situation before making a decision about how to behave. Rational thinking is based on accurate information and ideas, and leads to planned and positive decisions. Rational thinking leads to sensible behavior.
109. Rationalize. To make excuses for or explain away behavior, making it appear the behavior was okay or justifiable.
110. Relapse. A return to negative behaviors a person is trying to avoid. For a drug addict, it means returning to drug use. For a sexual offender, a relapse means returning to sexually abusive behaviors.
111. Relapse Prevention. The things we do to avoid falling back into old and destructive behavior that is experienced as harmful to us, and sometimes to others. In the case of sexually abusive behavior, relapse is always harmful to others.
112. Relapse Prevention Plan (sometimes also known as a "safe behavior plan"). An organized way to avoid relapse. A Relapse Prevention Plan includes steps that help us to understand when things are going wrong before they go wrong, and steps through which we can help ourselves and get help from others so that relapse doesn't follow. A carefully developed and written plan that helps you to avoid engaging in sexually abusive or sexually inappropriate behavior in the future.
113. Remorse. Feeling regretful, or sorry, about harmful or careless things we've done, or about positive things we haven't done.
114. Resources. Things, information, or people that can be used to support or help people, and that can be called on when needed.
115. Responsibility. A person's willingness to tell the truth, accept that behaviors are made by choice, and accept the consequences of choices.
116. Restitution. Making amends, making up or paying for some harm or damage you have caused, usually to the victims of your behaviors. Restitution, from the word "restore," is usually owed to the victims of your behaviors.
117. Risk Assessment. A way to measure your level of risk, reporting on how likely you are to engage again in sexually abusive or sexually inappropriate behavior in the future.
118. Risk Factor. Something that increases the chances that someone will be put into a bad situation, or something that increases the chances that someone will cause or experience some sort of harm.
119. Romantic. Involving feelings of closeness and connection, combined with physical attraction and sexual interest.
120. Safe Behavior Plan (sometimes also called a "relapse prevention plan"). A plan to help you to never again engage in sexually abusive or sexually inappropriate behavior.
121. Scripts. These are internalized and nearly automatic ways of thinking that often guide our behavior. Scripts allow us to act without thinking too hard, and can contain both positive and negative ideas about people and the world.
122. Seemingly Unimportant Decisions (SUDs). Choices and actions that seem trivial and unimportant, but are actually small steps that return you to a problem situation or behavior.
123. Self-Awareness. Having a sense of your own self, including your feelings, your thoughts, and your behaviors, as well as your personality and your sense of identity.
124. Self-Defeating. Personal behaviors that hurt, instead of help, our chances of success.
125. Self-Destructive. A description of the harm or injury caused by our behaviors to ourselves.
126. Self-Destructive Behavior. Behavior that is harmful to you, physically or mentally, and that also hurts your goals and interests.

127. Sequence. One thing follows another in a predictable order.
128. Sex Offender Registry. The state government list on which sexual offenders must be listed, although the requirements vary from state to state. Information about registered sexual offenders is available to the public.
129. Sexual Abuse. Another term for when a sexual offense has been committed. An act of sexual abuse may or may not involve legal charges, but it always involves a sexual act with someone against his or her will or with someone who can't give permission for sex.
130. Sexual Assault. The legal term that can apply to a number of unwanted sexual or sexually abusive behaviors, including rape.
131. Sexual Offenses. Behaviors that involve making someone engage in a sexual behavior against his or her will, having sexual contact with someone too young to give permission, or having sexual contact with someone who can't give permission for another reason (such as being drugged or asleep).
132. Sexualized Coping. This is an attempt to feel better and deal with things by using sexual behavior as a way to cope with problems, frustrations, disappointments, and difficulties.
133. Sexually Abusive Behavior. Any sexual behavior with another person that is abusive because, (a) the other person does not want to engage in sexual behaviors with you or be exposed to your sexual behaviors, (b) the other person is too young to engage in sexual behavior, or is at least three or more years younger than you. or, (c) the other person is not able to give permission (consent) for sexual behavior because of his or her age, mental abilities that don't allow him or her to make clear decisions about what is right or wrong, or because he or she is drunk, drugged, or unconscious (including being asleep).
134. Sexually Inappropriate Behavior. Behavior of a sexual nature that does not rise to the level of sexual abuse but is still unwanted by the other person, or sexual behavior that occurs in the wrong place or at the wrong time.
135. Social Skills. Abilities you use in your daily life that range from your personal hygiene to coping with difficult situations, knowing how to deal with other people, and conducting yourself in public.
136. Support Group/Network. A "network" or a connected group of people who are there to help, lend assistance, and support us when things are difficult or when we need an extra push.
137. Support. To give assistance and comfort to someone in difficulty or distress. Support and help are almost the same thing. People support you when they offer help, but people also support you when they help hold you up during difficult times. Support can hold us together when things are difficult for us. Support often makes all the difference between success and failure. Support helps us to overcome our weaknesses, build our strengths, and meet our goals.
138. Sympathy. Feeling sorry for another person, feeling support for another person.
139. Therapeutic Relationship. The important, strong, and trusting relationship built between you and your therapist as you both work together, to help bring about important changes in your life.
140. Thinking Errors. Ways of thinking that are based on inaccurate or mistaken ideas (sometimes called "cognitive distortions").
141. Thought. The ideas in our heads and the words we put onto our feelings and experiences.
142. Tolerate. To put up with something difficult or negative, such as an unpleasant feeling or thought.
143. Tone of Voice. Non-verbal communication that is conveyed through the way that someone speaks to others, including the sound or the volume of their voice, the use of sarcasm, or an attitude in their voice.
144. Treatment. The discussions, activities, and programs that help you change in ways that will help make you more successful and safer for others.
145. Treatment Goals. The things that you and your treatment team are working towards accomplishing, so that you can move towards being a person who is safe (to yourself and others), satisfied, and successful.
146. Trigger. An Event or circumstance that sets a dysfunctional behavioral cycle into motion.
147. Urge. A feeling that people have to do something right now, usually without further thought or consideration. An urge is similar to an "impulse" in which you act without thinking, or act on an urge.
148. Urge Control. Also known as "impulse control," involves the ability to not give in to an urge, an impulse, or a craving.
149. Value. Something meaningful to you, in which you place importance. Something that helps guide your decisions and the way you live your life.
150. Value System. A set or collection of values that help shape the things you do or think, or the way you live your life.
151. Victim. A person who has been harmed by another person or a situation. In sexual abuse, victims are people who are forced to have sex, tricked into a sexual interaction, or too young or otherwise unable to give permission for sex.
152. Victimization. The act of harming another person (making someone a victim) by taking advantage of him or her, taking control over the other person, or exploiting that person in some other way in order to meet your own needs and without any concern for the other person.
153. Voyeurism. Also known as "peeping," sneaking a look at people when they're getting undressed or are naked, or watching someone having sex, usually without their knowledge and without their consent.
154. Vulnerabilities. The qualities, tendencies, and reactions that can limit us by interfering with goal achievement, weaken us, or make us open to failure. It is important to recognize and face our vulnerabilities, not allow them to lead us to poor choices, and, as important, not allowing them to .stop us from making good decisions.
155. Warning Sign. Something that tells someone that a behavior of some kind is possibly problematic or unsafe. Feeling an urge, an impulse, or a craving are all examples of warning signs that tell you to think hard about whether the behavior you're considering is wise or safe. Warning signs are like red flags that pop up to warn or remind us about safety.

Workbook Tests

It is not possible to devise "tests" that will fit the goal of every clinician or program. The tests included in this appendix offer a simple method of testing, based on both description and definition, and can be used "as is" or as templates from which clinicians or programs may re-design tests that better fit their particular needs.

Stages of Accomplishment: Stage 1 Test

Youth: ______________________________ Test Date: ____________________

Treatment Staff: ______________________________ Test Sitting #: _____

Question Score: ___ Definitions Score: ___

Instructions

- On this test, there are 16 questions for you to answer. To pass the Stage 1 test you have to correctly answer 13 of these questions.
- There are also 20 words that you must provide definitions for. You have to provide correct definitions for 17 of these words.
- Take as much time as you need to answer these questions. You can use your Stage 1 workbook to help you, if needed.
- If you don't have the answer to a question, just skip the question or write that you don't know.
- Your clinician or another member of your treatment team will review your test when complete, and decide whether you've passed.
- If you don't pass the test, don't worry. You can go over the test with your clinician or another member of your treatment team. She or he will help you to understand any questions that you didn't understand or got wrong, and you can take the test again one week (7 days) later.

Test Questions

1. What does "confidentiality" mean? P__ F__

____

____

____

2. Do therapists always keep confidentiality? P__ F__

____

____

____

3. When might a therapist not keep confidentiality? P__ F__

____

____

____

4. How are "responsibility" and "choice" connected to one another? P__ F__

____

____

____

5. How do you know if someone's behavior is sexually abusive? P__ F__

____

____

____

Stage 1 Test

6. Give an example of taking responsibility. P__ F__

____

____

____

7. In your own words, what is denial? P__ F__

____

____

____

8. Name five of the guidelines for effective individual therapy. P__ F__

   1. ____________________________________
   2. ____________________________________
   3. ____________________________________
   4. ____________________________________
   5. ____________________________________

9. What are the first four steps in the twelve steps of treatment? P__ F__

   1. ____________________________________
   2. ____________________________________
   3. ____________________________________
   4. ____________________________________

10. Describe three of the "Five Rules to Live By." P__ F__

   1. ____________________________________
   2. ____________________________________
   3. ____________________________________

11. What makes a sexual act abusive? P__ F__

____

____

____

12. Describe six "rules" for participation in group therapy. P__ F__

   1. ____________________________________
   2. ____________________________________
   3. ____________________________________
   4. ____________________________________
   5. ____________________________________
   6. ____________________________________

13. How many therapists does it take to change light bulb, and why? P__ F__

It takes ____ therapists to change a light bulb, because ______________________________

____

14. What is an "I" Statement? P__ F__

____

____

____

15. What are the three elements of sexually abusive behavior? P__ F__

1. ____

2. ____

3. ____

16. What are "hands-on" sexual offenses? P__ F__

____

____

____

____

Definitions

Provide a definition for each of these words.

1. *Choice.* ____

____ P__ F__

2. *Coercion.* ____

____ P__ F__

3. *Consent.* ____

____ P__ F__

4. *Consequences.* ____

____ P__ F__

5. *Denial.* ____

____ P__ F__

6. *Equality.* ____

____ P__ F__

7. *Genuine.* ____

____ P__ F__

8. *Non-Consensual.* ____

____ P__ F__

9. *Perpetrator.* ____

____ P__ F__

10. *Personal Change.* ____

____ P__ F__

11. *Responsibility.* ____

____ P__ F__

12. *Restitution.* ____

____ P__ F__

13. *Sexually Abusive Behavior.* ____

____ P__ F__

14. *Sexually Inappropriate Behavior.* ____

____ P__ F__

15. *Sexual Offense.* ____

____ P__ F__

16. *Social Skills.* ____

____ P__ F__

17. *Support.* ____

____ P__ F__

18. *Treatment Goal.* ____

____ P__ F__

19. *Victim.* ____

____ P__ F__

20. *Victimization.* ____

____ P__ F__

Stage 1 Scoring

Questions		Correct	Incorrect
1.	Confidentiality	___	___
2.	Clinician will keep confidentiality	___	___
3.	When might clinician not keep confidentiality	___	___
4.	Responsibility and choice	___	___
5.	Is behavior sexually abusive	___	___
6.	Example of responsibility	___	___
7.	What is denial	___	___
8.	Five rules for individual therapy *(5 out of 5)*	___	___
9.	First four of twelve treatment steps *(4 out of 4)*	___	___
10.	Three of Five Rules to Live By *(3 out of 3)*	___	___
11.	What makes sexual act abusive	___	___
12.	Six rules for group therapy *(6 out of 6)*	___	___
13.	Therapists to change light bulb, and why	___	___
14.	"I" Statement	___	___
15.	Three elements of sexually abusive behavior *(3 out of 3)*	___	___
16.	Hands-on sexual offense	___	___

Total (13 to pass): ___

Definitions	Correct	Incorrect
1. Choice	__	__
2. Coercion	__	__
3. Consent	__	__
4. Consequences	__	__
5. Denial	__	__
6. Equality	__	__
7. Genuine	__	__
8. Non-Consensual	__	__
9. Perpetrator	__	__
10. Personal Change	__	__
11. Responsibility	__	__
12. Restitution	__	__
13. Sexually Abusive Behavior	__	__
14. Sexually Inappropriate Behavior	__	__
15. Sexual Offense	__	__
16. Social Skills	__	__
17. Support	__	__
18. Treatment Goal	__	__
19. Victim	__	__
20. Victimization	__	__

Total (17 to pass): __

Stage 1 Test

Stages of Accomplishment: Stage 2 Test

Youth: ______________________________ Test Date: ______________

Treatment Staff: ______________________ Test Sitting #: ____

Question Score: ___ Definitions Score: ___

Instructions

- On this test, there are 20 questions for you to answer. To pass the Stage 2 test you have to correctly answer 17 of these questions.
- There are also 20 words that you must provide definitions for. You have to provide correct definitions for 17 of these words.
- Take as much time as you need to answer these questions. You can use your Stage 2 workbook to help you, if needed.
- If you don't have the answer to a question, just skip the question or write that you don't know.
- Your clinician or another member of your treatment team will review your test when complete, and decide whether you've passed.
- If you don't pass the test, don't worry. You can go over the test with your clinician or another member of your treatment team. She or he will help you to understand any questions that you didn't understand or got wrong, and you can take the test again one week (7 days) later.

Test Questions

1. What is the difference between a vulnerability and a strength? P__ F__

____

____

____

2. Why are goals important? P__ F__

____

____

____

3. What does it mean to think rationally? P__ F__

____

____

____

5. How are our feelings like a weather vane? P__ F__

____

____

____

6. How is anger like a worm? P__ F__

____

____

____

Stage 2 Test

7. What does managing your feelings mean? P__ F__

____

____

____

8. What are three steps to understanding and managing behavior? P__ F__

1. ______________________________

2. ______________________________

3. ______________________________

9. Name six feelings. P__ F__

1. ______________ 4. ______________

2. ______________ 5. ______________

3. ______________ 6. ______________

10. What is healthy coping? P__ F__

____

____

____

11. Give an example of unhealthy coping. P__ F__

____

____

____

12. Describe four healthy coping mechanisms. P__ F__

1. ______________ 3. ______________

2. ______________ 4. ______________

13. How can beliefs and attitudes hurt other people? P__ F__

____

____

____

14. What is a value? P__ F__

____

____

____

15. Give three examples of values. P__ F__

1. ______________________________

2. ______________________________

3. ______________________________

16. What is a thinking error? P__ F__

____

____

____

17. Name the three types of thinking errors. P__ F__

1. ______________________________
2. ______________________________
3. ______________________________

18. Describe six types of thinking errors. P__ F__

1. ______________ 4. ______________
2. ______________ 5. ______________
3. ______________ 6. ______________

19. How can thinking errors be harmful? P__ F__

____

____

____

20. Describe a pro-social attitude and give one example. P__ F__

____

____

____

____

____

Definitions

Provide a definition for each of these words.

1. *Attitude.* ______________________________

______________________________ P__ F__

2. *Antisocial.* ______________________________

______________________________ P__ F__

3. *Cognitive distortion.* ______________________________

______________________________ P__ F__

4. *Dysfunctional.* ______________________________

______________________________ P__ F__

5. *Goal.* ______________________________

______________________________ P__ F__

6. *Healthy.* ______________________________

______________________________ P__ F__

Stage 2 Test

7. *Impulsive.* ____

____ P__ F__

8. *Internalize.* ____

____ P__ F__

9. *Irrational Thinking.* ____

____ P__ F__

10. *Manage.* ____

____ P__ F__

11. *Pro-social.* ____

____ P__ F__

12. *Rational Thinking.* ____

____ P__ F__

13. *Self-Defeating.* ____

____ P__ F__

14. *Strength.* ____

____ P__ F__

15. *Support Network.* ____

____ P__ F__

16. *Thinking Error.* ____

____ P__ F__

17. *Tolerate.* ____

____ P__ F__

18. *Urge.* ____

____ P__ F__

19. *Value.* ____

____ P__ F__

20. *Vulnerability.* ____

____ P__ F__

Stage 2 Scoring

Questions	Correct	Incorrect
1. Why are goals important	___	___
2. What does it mean to think rationally	___	___
3. How are our feelings like a weather vane	___	___
5. Why is anger like a worm	___	___
6. What does managing your feelings mean	___	___
7. Three steps to understanding and managing behavior *(3 out of 3)*	___	___
8. Name six feelings *(5 out of 6)*	___	___

9.	Healthy coping	___	___
10.	Example of unhealthy coping	___	___
11.	Describe four healthy coping mechanisms *(3 out of 4)*	___	___
12.	How can beliefs and attitudes hurt other people	___	___
13.	What is a value	___	___
14.	Three examples of values *(3 out of 3)*	___	___
15.	What is a thinking error	___	___
16.	Name the three groups of thinking errors *(3 out of 3)*	___	___
17.	Six types of thinking errors *(six out of six)*	___	___
18.	How can thinking errors be harmful	___	___
19.	Pro-social attitude, and one example	___	___
20.	Difference between a vulnerability and a strength	___	___

Total (17 to pass): ___

	Definitions	**Correct**	**Incorrect**
1.	Attitude	___	___
2.	Antisocial	___	___
3.	Cognitive distortion	___	___
4.	Dysfunctional	___	___
5.	Goal	___	___
6.	Healthy	___	___
7.	Impulsive	___	___
8.	Internalize	___	___
9.	Irrational Thinking	___	___
10.	Manage	___	___
11.	Pro-social	___	___
12.	Rational Thinking	___	___
13.	Self-Defeating	___	___
14.	Strength	___	___
15.	Support Network	___	___
16.	Thinking Error	___	___
17.	Tolerate	___	___
18.	Urge	___	___
19.	Value	___	___
20.	Vulnerability	___	___

Total (17 to pass): ___

Stage 2 Test

Stages of Accomplishment: Stage 3 Test

Youth: ______________________ Test Date: ______________

Treatment Staff: ______________________ Test Sitting #: ____

Question Score: ___ Definitions Score: ___

Instructions

- On this test, there are 20 questions for you to answer. To pass the Stage 3 test you have to correctly answer 17 of these questions.
- There are also 20 words that you must provide definitions for. You have to provide correct definitions for 17 of these words.
- Take as much time as you need to answer these questions. You can use your Stage 3 workbook to help you, if needed.
- If you don't have the answer to a question, just skip the question or write that you don't know.
- Your clinician or another member of your treatment team will review your test when complete, and decide whether you've passed.
- If you don't pass the test, don't worry. You can go over the test with your clinician or another member of your treatment team. She or he will help you to understand any questions that you didn't understand or got wrong, and you can take the test again one week (7 days) later.

Test Questions

1. Starting with the trigger, name the five points of a behavioral cycle. P__ F__

   1. ______________________

   2. ______________________

   3. ______________________

   4. ______________________

   5. ______________________

2. What is a dysfunctional behavioral cycle? P__ F__

   ____

   ____

   ____

3. Name the five phases of the dysfunctional behavioral cycle, and give a brief description of each phase. P__ F__

	Phase	*Description*
1.	__________	____________________
2.	__________	____________________
3.	__________	____________________
4.	__________	____________________
5.	__________	____________________

4. What does "high-risk situation" mean? P__ F__

____

____

____

5. Give three examples of things that might make something high-risk. P__ F__

   1. ____

   2. ____

   3. ____

6. What is PIG, and why is PIG a problem? P__ F__

____

____

____

7. What do we mean by a risk factor? P__ F__

____

____

____

8. What do we mean by a protective factor? P__ F__

____

____

____

9. What do we mean by a seemingly unimportant decision? P__ F__

____

____

____

10. Give two examples of seemingly unimportant decisions. P__ F__

    1. ____

    2. ____

11. Why might impulsive behavior be destructive to someone? P__ F__

____

____

____

12. Why are some forms of coping unsuccessful? P__ F__

____

____

____

Stage 3 Test

13. Give two examples of negative coping. P__ F__

1. ______________________________

2. ______________________________

14. What do we mean by sexualized coping? P__ F__

____

____

____

15. What is a behavior management plan? P__ F__

____

____

____

16. What is a relapse prevention plan? P__ F__

____

____

____

17. What is relapse? P__ F__

____

____

____

18. Name two goals of a relapse prevention plan. P__ F__

1. ______________________________

2. ______________________________

19. How might sexualized coping be related to sexually abusive behavior? P__ F__

____

____

____

20. What does "interrupting the cycle" mean, and why is it important to interrupt the cycle? P__ F__

____

____

____

Definitions

Provide a definition for each of these words.

1. *Behavior Management.* ______________________________

______________________________ P__ F__

2. *Consequences.* ______________________________

______________________________ P__ F__

3. *Coping.* ____

____ P__ F__

4. *Craving.* ____

____ P__ F__

5. *Denial.* ____

____ P__ F__

6. *Dysfunctional.* ____

____ P__ F__

7. *Dysfunctional Behaviors.* ____

____ P__ F__

8. *Empathy.* ____

____ P__ F__

9. *Impulse.* ____

____ P__ F__

10. *Interrupting the Cycle.* ____

____ P__ F__

11. *Lapse.* ____

____ P__ F__

12. *Minimization.* ____

____ P__ F__

13. *Narcissism.* ____

____ P__ F__

14. *Obstacle.* ____

____ P__ F__

15. *Relapse.* ____

____ P__ F__

16. *Relapse Prevention.* ____

____ P__ F__

17. *Sexualized Coping.* ____

____ P__ F__

18. *Trigger.* ____

____ P__ F__

19. *Urge.* ____

____ P__ F__

20. *Urge Control.* ____

____ P__ F__

Stage 3 Test

Stage 3 Scoring

Questions	Correct	Incorrect
1. Name the five points of a behavioral cycle *(5 out of 5)*.	___	___
2. What is dysfunctional behavioral cycle	___	___
3. Five phases of dysfunctional cycle, and description *(5 out of 5)*.	___	___
4. What does "high-risk situation" mean	___	___
5. Three examples of things that make high-risk.	___	___
6. What is PIG, and why is it a problem	___	___
7. What do we mean by risk factor	___	___
8. What do we mean by a protective factor	___	___
9. What do we mean by a seemingly unimportant decision	___	___
10. Two examples of seemingly unimportant decisions.	___	___
11. Why might impulsive behavior be destructive to someone	___	___
12. Why are some forms of coping unsuccessful	___	___
13. Two examples of negative coping.	___	___
14. What do we mean by sexualized coping	___	___
15. What is a behavior management plan	___	___
16. What is a relapse prevention plan	___	___
17. What is relapse	___	___
18. Three goals of a relapse prevention plan.	___	___
19. How is sexualized coping related to sexually abusive behavior	___	___
20. Define interrupting the cycle, and why is it important to interrupt	___	___

Total (17 to pass): ___

Definitions	Correct	Incorrect
1. Behavior Management.	___	___
2. Consequences	___	___
3. Coping	___	___
4. Craving.	___	___
5. Denial	___	___
6. Dysfunctional	___	___
7. Dysfunctional Behaviors	___	___
8. Empathy	___	___
9. Impulse.	___	___
10. Interrupting the Cycle	___	___
11. Lapse.	___	___
12. Minimization.	___	___
13. Narcissism.	___	___
14. Obstacle.	___	___
15. Relapse.	___	___
16. Relapse Prevention	___	___
17. Sexualized Coping.	___	___
18. Trigger.	___	___
19. Urge.	___	___
20. Urge Control.	___	___

Total (17 to pass): ___

Stages of Accomplishment: Stage 4 Test

Youth: ______________________________ Test Date: ______________

Treatment Staff: ______________________ Test Sitting #: ____

Question Score: ___ Definitions Score: ___

Instructions

- On this test, there are 20 questions for you to answer. To pass the Stage 4 test you have to correctly answer 17 of these questions.
- There are also 20 words that you must provide definitions for. You have to provide correct definitions for 17 of these words.
- Take as much time as you need to answer these questions. You can use your Stage 4 workbook to help you, if needed.
- If you don't have the answer to a question, just skip the question or write that you don't know.
- Your clinician or another member of your treatment team will review your test when complete, and decide whether you've passed.
- If you don't pass the test, don't worry. You can go over the test with your clinician or another member of your treatment team. She or he will help you to understand any questions that you didn't understand or got wrong, and you can take the test again one week (7 days) later.

Test Questions

1. What does taking perspective mean? *P__ F__*

   ____

   ____

   ____

2. Why is empathy an important relationship skill? *P__ F__*

   ____

   ____

   ____

3. What makes morality so important to relationships? *P__ F__*

   ____

   ____

   ____

4. What is victim clarification? *P__ F__*

   ____

   ____

   ____

5. Name four things we want to see in the perpetrator before victim clarification sessions take place. *P__ F__*

   1. ____________________ *2.* ____________________

   3. ____________________ *4.* ____________________

7. Describe four important elements of an apology letter. P__ F__

1. ______________________________

2. ______________________________

3. ______________________________

4. ______________________________

8. What does it mean to belong to a community? P__ F__

9. What is community learning? P__ F__

10. What is community service? P__ F__

11. How can people help build their communities? P__ F__

12. Why is communication such an important skill? P__ F__

13. Why is nonverbal communication important? P__ F__

14. What is active listening and why is it so important? P__ F__

15. Name six of the rules for effective communication. P__ F__

1. ______________________________

2. ______________________________

3. ____________________

4. ____________________

5. ____________________

6. ____________________

16. Describe four of the eight guidelines for giving positive feedback. P__ F__

1. ____________________

2. ____________________

3. ____________________

4. ____________________

17. What is an unhealthy relationship? P__ F__

____

____

____

18. Name six elements of a healthy relationship. P__ F__

1. ____________________

2. ____________________

3. ____________________

4. ____________________

5. ____________________

6. ____________________

19. Why are boundaries important to healthy relationships? P__ F__

____

____

____

20. Name the five rules for healthy relationships. P__ F__

1. ____________________

2. ____________________

3. ____________________

4. ____________________

5. ____________________

Definitions

Provide a definition for each of these words.

1. *Empathy.* ____________________

____________________ P__ F__

2. *Perspective.* ____________________

____________________ P__ F__

3. Remorse. ____
____ P__ F__

4. Morality. ____
____ P__ F__

5. Exploitation. ____
____ P__ F__

6. Clarification. ____
____ P__ F__

7. Community. ____
____ P__ F__

8. Community Service. ____
____ P__ F__

9. Community Learning. ____
____ P__ F__

10. Assumption. ____
____ P__ F__

11. Obstacle. ____
____ P__ F__

12. Nonverbal Communication. ____
____ P__ F__

13. Active Listening. ____
____ P__ F__

14. "I "Statement. ____
____ P__ F__

15. Feedback. ____
____ P__ F__

16. Judgmental. ____
____ P__ F__

17. Intimate. ____
____ P__ F__

18. Healthy Relationship. ____
____ P__ F__

19. Boundary. ____
____ P__ F__

20. Consensual. ____
____ P__ F__

Stage 4 Test

Stage 4 Scoring

Questions	Correct	Incorrect
1. What does taking perspective mean	___	___
2. Why is empathy an important relationship skill	___	___
3. What makes morality so important to relationships	___	___
4. What is victim clarification	___	___
5. Four things before victim clarification sessions take place *(4 out of 4)*	___	___
7. Four important elements of a apology letter *(4 out of 4)*	___	___
8. What does it mean to belong to a community	___	___
9. What is community learning	___	___
10. What is community service	___	___
11. How can people help build their communities	___	___
12. Why is communication such an important skills	___	___
13. Why is nonverbal communication important	___	___
14. What is active listening, and why is it so important	___	___
15. Six of the rules for effective communication *(6 out of 6)*	___	___
16. Four of the eight guidelines for giving positive feedback *(4 out of 4)*	___	___
17. What is an unhealthy relationship	___	___
18. Six elements of a healthy relationship *(6 out of 6)*	___	___
19. Why are boundaries important to healthy relationships	___	___
20. Five rules for healthy relationships *(5 out of 5)*	___	___

Total (17 to pass): ___

Definitions	Correct	Incorrect
1. Empathy	___	___
2. Perspective	___	___
3. Remorse	___	___
4. Morality	___	___
5. Exploitation	___	___
6. Clarification	___	___
7. Community	___	___
8. Community Service	___	___
9. Community Learning	___	___
10. Assumption	___	___
11. Obstacle	___	___
12. Nonverbal Communication	___	___
13. Active Listening	___	___
14. "I "Statement	___	___
15. Feedback	___	___
16. Judgmental	___	___
17. Intimate	___	___
18. Healthy Relationship	___	___
19. Boundary	___	___
20. Consensual	___	___

Total (17 to pass): ___

Stage 4 Test

References

Arkowitz, H., Westra, H.A., Miller, W.R., Rollnick, S. (Eds.) (2008). *Motivational interviewing in the treatment of psychological problems*. NY: Guilford Press.

Bordin, E.S. (1976). The generalizability of the psychoanalytical concept of the working alliance. *Psychotherapy: Theory, Research, and Practice, 16,* 252-260.

Castonguay, L.G., & Beutler, L.E. (2006). *Principles of therapeutic change that work.* NY: Oxford University Press.

Hubble, M.A., Duncan, B.L., & Miller, S.D. (1999). *The heart and soul of change: What works in therapy.* Washington, DC: American Psychological Association.

Lambert, M.J. (1992). Implications of outcome research for psychotherapy integration. In J.C. Norcross & M.R. Goldstein (Eds.), *Handbook of psychotherapy integration* (pp. 94-129). New York: Basic Books.

Lambert, M.J. & Bergin, A.E. (1993). The effectiveness of psychotherapy. In A.E. Bergin & S.L. Garfield (Eds). *Handbook of psychotherapy & behavior change* (4th ed.). (pp. 143-189). New York: John Wiley.

Letourneau, E.J., & Borduin, C.M. (2008) The effective treatment of juveniles who sexually offend: An ethical imperative. *Ethics and Behavior, 18,* 286-306.

Norcross, J.P. (2002). *Psychotherapy relationships that work: Therapist contributions and responsiveness to patients.* New York: Oxford University Press.

Wilbourne, P.L., & Levensky, E.R. (2006). Enhancing client motivation to change. In W. O'Donohue, N.A. Cummings, & J.L. Cummings (Eds.), *Clinical strategies for becoming a master psychotherapist* (pp. 11-36). Amsterdam, Netherlands: Elsevier. xi, 352 pp.

Ward, T., Polaschek, D.L.L., & Beech, A.R. (2006). *Theories of sexual offending.* Chicester, England: John Wiley & Sons.

Yates, P.M. (2007). Taking the leap: Abandoning relapse prevention and applying the self-regulation model to the treatment of sexual offenders. In D.S. Prescott (Ed.), *Knowledge and practice: Challenges in the treatment and supervision of sexual abusers* (pp. 143-174). Oklahoma City, OK: Wood'N'Barnes.

The NEARI Press
New England Adolescent Research Institute
70 North Summer Street
Holyoke, MA 01040
Phone 888.632.7412
www.neari.com

Assessing Youth Who Have Sexually Abused: A Primer
by David S. Prescott, LICSW (2007).
NEARI Press. Paperback, 98 pages.
ISBN# 978-1-929657-27-8

Current Perspectives: Working with Sexually Aggressive Youth and Youth with Sexual Behavior Problems
by R. E. Longo & D. S. Prescott (Editors)(2006).
NEARI Press. Hardcover, 720 pages.
ISBN# 978-1-929657-26-1

Enhancing Empathy
by Robert E. Longo and Laren Bays (1999).
NEARI Press. Paperback, 77 pages.
ISBN# 978-1-929657-04-9

Evolving Residential Work with Children and Families
by James R. Harris, Jr. (2009).
NEARI Press. Paperback, 159 pages.
ISBN# 978-1-929657-36-0

Growing Beyond: A Workbook for Teenage Girls
by Susan L. Robinson (2002).
NEARI Press. Paperback, 216 pages.
ISBN# 978-1-929657-17-9

Growing Beyond Treatment Manual: A Workbook for Sexually Abusive Teenage Girls
by Susan L. Robinson (2002).
NEARI Press. Paperback, 42 pages.
ISBN# 978-1-929657-15-5

Lessons from the Lion's Den: Therapeutic Management of Children in Psychiatric Hospitals and Treatment Centers
by Nancy S. Cotton, Ph.D. (2005).
NEARI Press. Paperback, 354 pages.
ISBN# 978-1-929657-24-7

Men & Anger: Understanding and Managing Your Anger
by Murray Cullen and Robert E. Longo (1996).
NEARI Press. Paperback, 125 pages.
ISBN# 978-1-929657-12-4

Moving Beyond Sexually Abusive Behavior: A Relapse Prevention Curriculum
by Thomas F. Leversee (2002).
NEARI Press. Paperback, 88 pages.
ISBN# 978-1-929657-16-2

Moving Beyond: Relapse Prevention Student Manual
by Thomas F. Leversee (2002).
NEARI Press. Paperback, 52 pages.
ISBN# 1-929657-18-6

New Hope For Youth: Experiential Exercises for Children & Adolescents
by Robert E. Longo & Deborah P. Longo (2003).
NEARI Press. Paperback,150 pages.
ISBN# 978-1-929657-20-9

Paths To Wellness
by Robert E. Longo (2001).
NEARI Press. Paperback, 144 pages.
ISBN#1-929657-13-1

Paths To Wellness en Español!
by Robert E. Longo (2001).
NEARI Press. Paperback, 144 pages.
ISBN# 978-1-929657-31-5

Promoting Healthy Childhood Development Today
by James R. Harris, Jr. (2007).
NEARI Press. Paperback, 106 pages.
ISBN# 978-1-929657-30-8

Responsibility And Self-Management: A Client Workbook of Skills to Learn
by Jack Apsche and Jerry L. Jennings (2007).
NEARI Press. Paperback, 216 pages.
ISBN# 978-1-929657-29-2

Responsibility And Self-Management: A Clinician's Manual and Guide for Case Conceptualization
by Jack Apsche and Jerry L. Jennings (2007).
NEARI Press. Paperback, 118 pages.
ISBN# 978-1-929657-28-5

Smoothies For The Brain: Brain-Based Strategies To Defuse Behavior Problems in the Classroom
by Penny Cuninggim and Shannon Chabot, (2008).
NEARI Press. Paperback, 48 pages.
ISBN# 978-1-929657-35-3

Strong at the Broken Places: Building Resiliency in Survivors of Trauma
by Linda T. Sanford (2005).
NEARI Press. Paperback, 208 pages.
ISBN# 978-1-929657-25-4

The Safe Workbook for Youth: New Choices for a Healthy Lifestyle
by John McCarthy and Kathy MacDonald (2001).
NEARI Press. Paperback, 210 pages.
ISBN# 978-1-929657-14-8

Stages of Accomplishment
by Phil Rich (2009).
NEARI Press. Paperback.
Clinician's Manual
ISBN#: 978-1-929657-41-4
Introduction to Treatment, Vol I
ISBN#: 978-1-929657-37-7
Understanding Yourself, Vol II
ISBN#: 978-1-929657-38-4
Understanding Dysfunctional Behavior, Vol III
ISBN#: 978-1-929657-39-1
Hitting the Target: Making Change Permanent, Vol IV
ISBN#: 978-1-929657-40-7

The Thursday Group
by PeggyElen Kleinleder and Kimber Everson (2009). NEARI Press. Paperback, 280 pages.
ISBN# 978-1-929657-44-5

Try and Make Me! Power Struggles: A Book of Strategies for Adults Who Live and Work with Angry Kids
by Penny Cuninggim (2003).
NEARI Press. Paperback, 112 pages.
ISBN# 978-1-929657-23-0

Using Conscience as a Guide: Enhancing Sex Offender Treatment in the Moral Domain
by Niki Delson (2003).
NEARI Press. Paperback, 102 pages.
ISBN# 978-1-929657-22-3

Using Conscience as a Guide: Student Manual
by Niki Delson (2003).
NEARI Press. Paperback, 50 pages.
ISBN# 978-1-929657-19-3

Who Am I and Why Am I In Treatment?
by Robert E. Longo with Laren Bays (2000).
NEARI Press. Paperback, 85 pages.
ISBN# 978-1-929657-01-8

Why Did I Do It Again & How Can I Stop?
by Robert E. Longo with Laren Bays (1999).
NEARI Press. Paperback, 192 pages.
ISBN# 978-1-929657-11-7

For prices and shipping information, or to order, please call: **888.632.7412**
Find us online at: **www.neari.com**